STRATEGIES TO LIMIT SUGAR-SWEETENED BEVERAGE CONSUMPTION IN YOUNG CHILDREN

PROCEEDINGS OF A WORKSHOP

Nancy Konopasek and Meghan Quirk, *Rapporteurs*

Food and Nutrition Board

Health and Medicine Division

The National Academies of
SCIENCES · ENGINEERING · MEDICINE

THE NATIONAL ACADEMIES PRESS
Washington, DC
www.nap.edu

THE NATIONAL ACADEMIES PRESS 500 Fifth Street, NW Washington, DC 20001

This activity was supported by contracts between the National Academy of Sciences and The California Endowment, Chobani Foundation, and Robert Wood Johnson Foundation. Any opinions, findings, conclusions, or recommendations expressed in this publication do not necessarily reflect the views of any organization or agency that provided support for the project.

International Standard Book Number-13: 978-0-309-46632-5
International Standard Book Number-10: 0-309-46632-6
Digital Object Identifier: https://doi.org/10.17226/24910

Additional copies of this publication are available for sale from the National Academies Press, 500 Fifth Street, NW, Keck 360, Washington, DC 20001; (800) 624-6242 or (202) 334-3313; http://www.nap.edu.

Printed in the United States of America

Suggested citation: National Academies of Sciences, Engineering, and Medicine. 2017. *Strategies to limit sugar-sweetened beverage consumption in young children: Proceedings of a workshop*. Washington, DC: The National Academies Press. doi: https://doi.org/10.17226/24910.

The National Academies of

SCIENCES • ENGINEERING • MEDICINE

The National Academy of Sciences was established in 1863 by an Act of Congress, signed by President Lincoln, as a private, nongovernmental institution to advise the nation on issues related to science and technology. Members are elected by their peers for outstanding contributions to research. Dr. Marcia McNutt is president.

The National Academy of Engineering was established in 1964 under the charter of the National Academy of Sciences to bring the practices of engineering to advising the nation. Members are elected by their peers for extraordinary contributions to engineering. Dr. C. D. Mote, Jr., is president.

The National Academy of Medicine (formerly the Institute of Medicine) was established in 1970 under the charter of the National Academy of Sciences to advise the nation on medical and health issues. Members are elected by their peers for distinguished contributions to medicine and health. Dr. Victor J. Dzau is president.

The three Academies work together as the **National Academies of Sciences, Engineering, and Medicine** to provide independent, objective analysis and advice to the nation and conduct other activities to solve complex problems and inform public policy decisions. The National Academies also encourage education and research, recognize outstanding contributions to knowledge, and increase public understanding in matters of science, engineering, and medicine.

Learn more about the National Academies of Sciences, Engineering, and Medicine at **www.nationalacademies.org**.

PLANNING COMMITTEE ON STRATEGIES TO LIMIT SUGAR-SWEETENED BEVERAGE CONSUMPTION IN YOUNG CHILDREN[1]

KAREN WEBER CULLEN (*Chair*), Professor, Pediatrics-Nutrition, Children's Nutrition Research Center, Baylor College of Medicine
LEANN BIRCH, William P. Flatt Professor, Department of Foods and Nutrition, University of Georgia
ESA DAVIS, Associate Professor Medicine, Clinical and Translational Science, Director, University of Pittsburgh Medical Center Tobacco Treatment Service, University of Pittsburgh
BARBARA DEVANEY, Senior Fellow, Mathematica Policy Research
CHRISTINA ECONOMOS, Professor and the New Balance Chair in Childhood Nutrition, Friedman School of Nutrition Science and Policy and Medical School, Tufts University, and Co-Founder and Director, ChildObesity180
BRIAN ELBEL, Associate Professor, Population Health and Health Policy, School of Medicine and Wagner School of Public Service, New York University
TRACY FOX, President, Food, Nutrition and Policy Consultants, LLC
BARRY POPKIN, W.R. Kenan, Jr. Distinguished Professor Gillings School of Global Public Health, Director Global Food Research Program, University of North Carolina at Chapel Hill
ANNA MARIA SIEGA-RIZ, Professor of Nursing and Associate Dean for Research, School of Nursing; jointly appointed in Public Health Sciences and Obstetrics and Gynecology, University of Virginia

Health and Medicine Division Staff

MEGHAN QUIRK, Project Director
MEREDITH YOUNG, Senior Program Assistant
ANN YAKTINE, Director, Food and Nutrition Board

[1] The National Academies of Sciences, Engineering, and Medicine's planning committees are solely responsible for organizing the workshop, identifying topics, and choosing speakers. The responsibility for the published Proceedings of a Workshop rests with the workshop rapporteurs and the institution.

Reviewers

This Proceedings of a Workshop was reviewed in draft form by individuals chosen for their diverse perspectives and technical expertise. The purpose of this independent review is to provide candid and critical comments that will assist the National Academies of Sciences, Engineering, and Medicine in making each published proceedings as sound as possible and to ensure that it meets the institutional standards for quality, objectivity, evidence, and responsiveness to the charge. The review comments and draft manuscript remain confidential to protect the integrity of the process.

We thank the following individuals for their review of this proceedings:

STEPHEN DANIELS, University of Colorado School of Medicine
ANNE FERREE, Alliance for a Healthier Generation
RACHEL JOHNSON, University of Vermont
BERNADETTE MARRIOTT, Medical University of South Carolina
BARBARA O. SCHNEEMAN, University of California, Davis (Emeritus)

Although the reviewers listed above provided many constructive comments and suggestions, they were not asked to endorse the content of the proceedings nor did they see the final draft before its release. The review of this proceedings was overseen by **HUGH H. TILSON,** University of North Carolina at Chapel Hill. He was responsible for making certain that an independent examination of this proceedings was carried out in accordance with standards of the National Academies and that all review comments were carefully considered. Responsibility for the final content rests entirely with the rapporteurs and the National Academies.

Contents

Acronyms and Abbreviations

AAP	American Academy of Pediatrics
BMI	body mass index
BRFSS	Behavioral Risk Factor Surveillance System
CACFP	Child and Adult Care Food Program
CDC	Centers for Disease Control and Prevention
CFBAI	Children's Food and Beverage Advertising Initiative
CFOC	Caring for Our Children
CHOICES	Childhood Obesity Intervention Cost-Effectiveness Study
COPE	Community Outreach and Patient Empowerment
DGA	*Dietary Guidelines for Americans*
DGAC	Dietary Guidelines Advisory Committee
DNPAO	Division of Nutrition, Physical Activity, and Obesity
ECE	early care and education
FITS	Feeding Infants and Toddlers Study
HER	Healthy Eating Research
IFPS II	Infant Feeding Practices Study II
IOM	Institute of Medicine

NAP SACC	Nutrition and Physical Activity Self-Assessment for Child Care
NB3	Notah Begay III (Foundation)
NCCOR	National Collaborative on Childhood Obesity Research
NHANES	National Health and Nutrition Examination Survey
NYC DOHMH	New York City Department of Health and Mental Hygiene
QRIS	Quality Rating and Improvement System
RWJF	Robert Wood Johnson Foundation
SNAP	Supplemental Nutrition Assistance Program
SNAP-Ed	Supplemental Nutrition Assistance Program Education
SSB	sugar-sweetened beverage
USDA	U.S. Department of Agriculture
WHO	World Health Organization
WIC	Special Supplemental Nutrition Program for Women, Infants, and Children

1

Introduction and Workshop Overview

On June 21–22, 2017, the Food and Nutrition Board of the National Academies of Sciences, Engineering, and Medicine convened A Workshop on Strategies to Limit Sugar-Sweetened Beverage Consumption in Young Children: Evaluation of Federal, State, and Local Policies and Programs,[1,2] in Washington, DC. As guided by the Statement of Task (see Box 1-1), the workshop had five objectives:

1. Provide an overview of current and emerging strategies to reduce consumption of sugar-sweetened beverages by young children 0 to 5 years of age and explore the evidence on effectiveness;
2. Contextualize the strategies by broadly considering patterns and trends in beverage consumption, and specifically sugar-sweetened beverage consumption, in U.S. children;

[1] The planning committee's role was limited to planning the workshop, and this Proceedings of a Workshop was prepared by the workshop rapporteurs as a factual summary of what occurred at the workshop. Statements, recommendations, and opinions expressed are those of individual presenters and participants, and are not necessarily endorsed or verified by the National Academies of Sciences, Engineering, and Medicine, and they should not be construed as reflecting any group consensus.

[2] For consistency of language, the term *sugar-sweetened beverages* will be used throughout this Proceedings of a Workshop in lieu of other terms and abbreviations used by the speakers and moderators (e.g., *sugary drinks*, *SSBs*). A definition of sugar-sweetened beverages was not established for this workshop. Instead, speakers were asked to include in their presentations an explanation of the beverages to which they were referring when using the phrase. Unless otherwise noted, speakers discussed 100 percent fruit juice as a category separate from sugar-sweetened beverages.

BOX 1-1
Statement of Task

An ad hoc committee will plan a 1.5-day workshop that explores evidence from federal, state, local, and tribal policies, institutional policies affecting early care and education facilities, health care systems, food manufacturers and retailers, and programs currently in place on efforts to reduce consumption of sugar-sweetened beverages by children from 0 to 5 years of age. The workshop topics will include consideration of the prevalence and patterns of sugar-sweetened beverage consumption among the target age groups, development of taste preferences, the influence of sugar-sweetened beverage marketing practices aimed at young children on consumption of sugar-sweetened beverages, and the influence of social equity and health disparity, such as lifestyle, income, ethnicity, and place of residence on the effectiveness of efforts to reduce sugar-sweetened beverage consumption. Topics explored in the workshop will also include modeling policy and program effectiveness. A workshop-in-brief document and a workshop proceedings will be produced to summarize key messages from the workshop. Following the workshop, a planning meeting will be held to discuss stakeholder perspectives on the workshop topics, as well as interest in developing a pathway to move the field forward and the role that the National Academies could play in such an effort.

3. Examine current guidelines for beverage intake applicable to children 5 years of age and younger;
4. Explore the role of industry in sugar-sweetened beverage intake in young children; and
5. Identify where knowledge gaps and opportunities exist to inform future policies, programs, and strategies.

This Proceedings of a Workshop summarizes the presentations and discussions that took place over the course of the workshop.[3] This proceedings also expands on the key points highlighted in the Proceedings of a Workshop—in Brief (NASEM, 2017). It is not intended to be a comprehensive summary of the topic. Furthermore, citations herein correspond to those presented on speaker's slides and explicitly referred to during discussions, and do not constitute a comprehensive reference list on any of the subjects covered during the workshop. A bibliography of references used to inform workshop planning, provided as a handout at the workshop, is presented in Appendix C.

[3] Materials from the workshop, including presentations and videos, can be found at http://nationalacademies.org/hmd/Activities/Nutrition/StrategiesToLimitSSBConsumptioninYoungChildren/2017-JUN-21.aspx (accessed November 13, 2017).

ORGANIZATION OF THIS PROCEEDINGS OF A WORKSHOP

The organization of this Proceedings of a Workshop parallels the workshop agenda. This chapter provides an overview of the objectives and scope of the workshop, along with welcoming and opening remarks. Chapter 2 summarizes Session 1 presentations and discussions. Speakers provided context for the policies and programs by presenting prevalence and trends in beverage intake, discussing the potential cost-effectiveness of different strategies, and describing considerations related to drinking water. Chapter 3 summarizes Session 2 presentations on the scientific report of the 2015 Dietary Guidelines Advisory Committee and the guidelines from the American Academy of Pediatrics. Chapter 4 summarizes Session 3, in which speakers discussed a wide range of strategies that have been implemented at different levels throughout the United States. Chapter 5 summarizes Session 4 presentations, which explored programs and policies that could potentially be scaled up. Chapter 6 summarizes Session 5, in which presenters considered how industry has contributed to current consumption patterns and approaches industry is taking to reduce sugar-sweetened beverage consumption in young children. Chapter 7 captures an invited reflection on the workshop in Session 6, along with a panel discussion on evidence gaps and research needs that exist and possible opportunities to fill such gaps. References cited throughout this proceedings follow Chapter 7. The workshop agenda is presented in Appendix A. Biographical sketches of the speakers and session moderators are presented in Appendix B. A bibliography of references used to inform workshop planning is presented in Appendix C.

WELCOMING REMARKS

To open the workshop, Karen Weber Cullen, professor of pediatrics-nutrition with Children's Nutrition Research Center at the Baylor College of Medicine and chair of the planning committee, explained that the workshop agenda was developed by considering a day in the life of a young child. She noted that there are various settings in which someone makes a decision to offer a child a beverage and that a number of influences have the potential to affect the decision for the child to be served or to consume a sugar-sweetened beverage.

Discussing the format of the workshop, Cullen briefly explained the facilitated discussion format. Audience members were asked to record their questions for speakers on index cards or submit their questions via the webcast platform. Moderators were to use the audience questions to guide the discussion portion of the session.

OPENING REMARKS FROM THE WORKSHOP SPONSORS

After Cullen's welcome, a speaker from each of the three workshop sponsors provided brief opening remarks, describing the interest of their respective organizations in exploring the current landscape of national, state, tribal, and local strategies to limit sugar-sweetened beverage consumption in young children.

Tina Kauh, Research-Evaluation-Learning senior program officer at the Robert Wood Johnson Foundation (RWJF), began by explaining that her organization "has a vision for a nation that lives by a culture of health in which everyone in a diverse society has the opportunity to lead healthy lives, now and for generations to come." Healthy Children, Healthy Weight—one component of RWJF's approach to achieving its vision—is guided by the recognition that children need environments that foster health and that families should have the chance to provide such an environment to their children. Kauh explained that many children in the United States do not have the necessities needed to support their physical, social, and emotional development, which she noted are elements of health that begin developing early in life. Accordingly, RWJF considers health promotion in early childhood and health equity to be major priorities. Kauh explained how limiting sugar-sweetened beverage consumption among young children aligns with these priorities. She noted that by 2 years of age, approximately one in three children consumes sugar-sweetened beverages on a given day, and that sugar-sweetened beverages contribute approximately 100 calories per day to the diets of children 2 to 5 years of age. Disparities in intake also exist, such as greater sugar-sweetened beverage consumption among black children and children from families with lower socioeconomic status. Kauh stated that RWJF views safe drinking water as the healthiest beverage option for young children and suggested that increasing drinking water intake could be one mechanism for decreasing sugar-sweetened beverage intake. Recognizing that young children interact with a variety of caregivers—parents, teachers, child care providers—Kauh explained that RWJF will be working over the next several years to identify and support policy opportunities that can potentially improve the health and well-being of young children in settings where they spend much of their time.

Judi Larsen, program manager for The California Endowment, provided a brief overview of her organization. With priorities that include prevention and racial equity, The California Endowment works with a variety of leaders throughout the state of California to support building healthier communities. Larsen explained that The California Endowment's work seeks to operate through collective, rather than individual, action. As such, support is given to grassroots organizations and leaders. The California Endowment has worked in the area of limiting sugar-sweetened beverage consumption for 20 years, and has been "deliberate and intentional about making sure that water is readily available and free." Larsen noted that her organization's efforts on this topic have included evaluating the retail environment, developing strong messaging and communications, and working in a collective manner. Based on its experience, which included supporting the 1995 efforts to fluoridate the public water systems in California, The California Endowment recognizes the importance of understanding the community context. "We feel really strongly that a more explicit focus on racial equity creates more local ownership," said Larsen, noting that change in policies and practices can arise from pressure from the local community and local leadership. Larsen concluded her remarks by suggesting that there are opportunities to better align initiatives to improve drinking water access and efforts to limit sugar-sweetened beverage consumption.

Robert Post, senior director at the Chobani Nutrition Center and advisor to the Chobani Foundation, explained that the Chobani Foundation supports efforts that improve access to healthier food options, empower better food choices, and promote health, wellness, sports, and fitness in communities in Idaho, New York, and throughout the United States. From such work, the Chobani Foundation has come to recognize that families, seeking to make the best choices for their children's health, "want to know all the options for replacing empty calories [sugar-sweetened beverages] provide, and that means nutrient-dense beverages and foods and water," said Post. He stated that "there are many pieces of the puzzle to assess policies and programs to limit [sugar-sweetened beverages]." The Chobani Foundation's experience has revealed the importance of pragmatic and actionable policies and programs. Recognizing that the context of the entire diet needs to be considered, Post presented evidence from the *2015–2020 Dietary Guidelines for Americans* (HHS/USDA, 2015a) showing that children are consuming too many added sugars and too few nutrient-dense foods. Post wondered if programs and policies are leading to displacement of nutrient-deficient calories with nutrient-dense calories and whether they are incentivizing innovation and renovation to create more nutrient-dense beverages in the food sector to meet needs. He offered that dietary shifts require individuals to replace less healthy choices, which requires a "how to" approach showing simple shifts that can improve dietary quality and may be able to "stick" over the long run without banning or excluding certain foods. Citing Zheng et al. (2015), Post noted that displacing sugar-sweetened beverages with milk and water in children's diets is inversely associated with the development of obesity. As such, he suggested that dietary shifts from options of low-nutrient density to high-nutrient density are needed to improve dietary intake quality.

Post underscored the need for policies and programs that have evidence of working in real-world settings. He presented evidence for nutrition education approaches, policy systems, and environmental approaches that emphasize the concept of nutrient-density to fill the gap created in reducing sugar-sweetened beverage consumption (Anzman-Frasca et al., 2015; Bender et al., 2013; Goldberg et al., 2015; Kenney et al., 2015a; Raynor et al., 2012; Silver et al., 2017; Wang et al., 2012; Wright et al., 2015). Post pointed to evidence that sugar-sweetened beverage consumption is associated with poor diet quality and other adverse health behaviors (Arsenault et al., 2017; Burgermaster et al., 2017; Piernas et al., 2015) and noted that food pattern modeling can be used to assess dietary effects of meeting recommended intake levels (Britten et al., 2012). He concluded that in order to understand the effects of reducing, limiting, or replacing sugar-sweetened beverages from children's diets, each of which has unique nutritional effects, behavior in the context of the whole dietary pattern has to be considered.

2

Setting the Stage

To begin the first session, moderator Leann Birch, William P. Flatt Professor at the University of Georgia, noted that the human diet begins as a single drink—milk—and progressively becomes more varied, a transition that is relatively complete by the time a child reaches 2 years of age. It is during this transformational period that infants and young children learn how and what to eat. What is learned stems from the home setting and the family environment, and depends on a variety of factors, including "culture, ethnicity, socioeconomic status, feeding practices, and what foods happen to be available," said Birch. "We learn to associate foods with particular contexts, consequences, and with other flavors, and we watch others eat and we learn that way as well," she added. Repeated exposure to foods, drinks, and flavors is generally needed for an infant to gain familiarity and develop preferences. The liking for the taste of sweet, however, is unique. As an unlearned response, Birch continued, the preference for sweet serves as "an unconditioned stimulus for ingestion" that leads to an endogenous opioid release and can have an analgesic effect.

Drawing on points made in a commentary by Giddings and Mennella (2016), Birch indicated that the widespread availability of sweet in the food supply, coupled with the innate preference for the taste, has made young children susceptible to displacing other foods in the diet with items that are sweet. Putting her remarks in context of the workshop, Birch stated "This is what [we are] up against if you want [children] to drink water instead of sugar-sweetened beverages."

To provide a foundation for the strategies, policies, and programs discussed throughout the workshop, the session continued with presentations from four speakers. Anna Maria Siega-Riz, professor at the University of Virginia, and Mary Story, professor at Duke University, each discussed prevalence and trends in beverage intake among young children and highlighted disparities in sugar-sweetened beverage intake. Steven Gortmaker, professor of the practice of health sociology at the Harvard T.H. Chan School of Public Health, then described the estimated cost-effectiveness and projected health effect of three strategies to limit sugar-sweetened beverage intake in young children. Finally, Christina Hecht, senior policy advisor at the University of California Nutrition Policy Institute, provided an overview of considerations related to the safety, access, and promotion of drinking water. A facilitated discussion with all four session speakers followed the presentations.

PREVALENCE, TRENDS, AND DISPARITIES IN BEVERAGE INTAKE AMONG YOUNG CHILDREN

To provide insight into the current beverage intake levels, patterns, trends, and population group differences, Siega-Riz first presented evidence from two recent publications that used 2005–2012 National Health and Nutrition Examination Survey (NHANES) data on the beverage consumption of children from 0 to 23.9 months of age (Grimes et al., 2015; Miles and Siega-Riz, 2017). Story then discussed similar analyses of data of children 0 to 47.9 months of age from the Feeding Infants and Toddlers Study (FITS) 2016.

Findings from NHANES for Children 0 to 23.9 Months of Age[1]

Infant formula, human milk, and infant foods are the primary foods consumed by infants from 0 to 5.9 months of age, providing 99.3 percent of daily total energy intake (Grimes et al., 2015). The food sources contributing to total energy intake are more varied for infants 6 to 11.9 months of age. Siega-Riz noted that one of the first sweet beverages introduced to young children is 100 percent fruit juice. She explained that 6 percent of infants 0 to 5.9 months of age consume 100 percent fruit juice, a proportion that increases to approximately 38 percent among infants 6 to 11.9 months of age and 57 percent among children 12 to 23.9 months of age (Grimes et al., 2015). In addition to consumption becoming more prevalent, 100 percent fruit juice also contributes to a greater proportion of total energy intake with increasing age. One hundred percent fruit juice accounts for approximately 1.5 percent of total energy intake among infants 6 to 11.9 months of age and 5.9 percent among children 12 to 23.9 months of age

[1] This section summarizes information presented by Anna Maria Siega-Riz.

(Grimes et al., 2015). Furthermore, 100 percent juice is the fifth largest contributor to intake of total sugars among infants 6 to 11.9 months of age and the second largest contributor to intake of total sugars among children 12 to 23.9 months of age. Compared to 2005–2008, the overall prevalence of 100 percent fruit juice intake in 2009–2012 decreased among infants 0 to 5.9 and 6 to 11.9 months of age (Miles and Siega-Riz, 2017).

For context, Siega-Riz showed that prevalence of breastmilk, formula, and cow's milk intake among children 0 to 23.9 months of age remained relatively stable between 2005–2008 and 2009–2012 (Miles and Siega-Riz, 2017).

Siega-Riz then discussed sugar-sweetened beverages, which she defined as "carbonated soda, fruit-flavored drinks, sports drinks, [and] presweetened tea or other beverages." Approximately 1 percent of infants 0 to 5.9 months of age consume such beverages, with the proportion increasing to approximately 6 percent among infants 6 to 11.9 months of age and 32 percent among children 12 to 23.9 months of age (Grimes et al., 2015). Among children 12 to 23.9 months of age, sugar-sweetened beverages contribute 3.1 percent of total energy intake (Grimes et al., 2015). Siega-Riz acknowledged that the contribution of sugar-sweetened beverages to intake of total sugars among infants 6 to 11.9 months of age is small, but such beverages are the fourth largest contributor to intake of total sugars among children 12 to 23.9 months of age. Although there was no change in the overall prevalence in sugar-sweetened beverage consumption among children 6 to 23.9 months of age between 2005–2008 and 2009–2012, the prevalence of intake among Mexican-American children appears to be decreasing, largely attributed to reductions in soda intake (Miles and Siega-Riz, 2017). Fruit-flavored drink consumption did not significantly change in the overall sample or for any of the evaluated population groups between 2005–2008 and 2009–2012. Siega-Riz noted, however, that more non-Hispanic black children and Mexican-American children 6 to 23.9 months of age consume fruit-flavored drinks as compared to their non-Hispanic white counterparts.

Findings from FITS for Children 0 to 47.9 Months of Age[2]

FITS 2016 is a national, cross-sectional survey of parents and caregivers of U.S. infants, toddlers, and preschool-age children sponsored and funded by Nestlé Research and designed and carried out by RTI International, explained Story. Conducted in 2002, 2008, and 2016, FITS aims to collect data on infant feeding practices, nutrient intakes, food intakes, dietary patterns, and lifestyle behaviors. Dietary intake data are collected via a 24-

[2] This section summarizes information presented by Mary Story.

hour recall, with a subsample of participants providing two 24-hour recalls. The overall sample for FITS 2016, which consisted of 3,234 households with at least one child younger than 48 months, "reflects the geographic and sociodemographic diversity of the [United States]," described Story.

Analyses of FITS 2016 data indicate that a dietary shift occurs around 12 months of age, and, during this time, sweets and snacks begin to play an increasing role in the diet. Sweets and snacks contribute 9 percent of total energy intake among children 12 to 14.9 months of age, a proportion that progressively increases to 19 percent of total energy intake among children 36 to 47.9 months of age. Expressed as energy per capita, children 36 to 47.9 months of age consume approximately 224 calories from sweets per day. Story noted that 100 percent juice does not follow the same trend across age groups, as it contributes a relatively consistent 4 to 5 percent of total energy intake among older infants, toddlers, and preschool-age children.

After providing the context of total dietary intake of children 0 to 47.9 months of age, Story presented analyses specifically exploring beverage intake. She showed that water and milk are the most commonly consumed beverages among young children in this age range. Story highlighted two issues concerning milk intake. First, evidence from FITS 2016 suggests that there are infants being introduced to cow's milk before the recommended age of 12 months. Furthermore, approximately 15 to 20 percent of children 12 months of age and older did not consume any milk on the day of the survey, which Story indicated has implications for diet quality.

Story defined the category of sugar-sweetened beverages as "soft drinks, fruit-flavored drinks, teas and coffee, sports drinks, and other drinks, such as caloric flavored water or energy drinks." She noted the definition did not include flavored milk and 100 percent fruit juice. Evidence from FITS 2016 shows the proportion of children consuming sugar-sweetened beverages increased with increasing age. Approximately 1 percent of children 0 to 5.9 months of age reportedly consumed any sugar-sweetened beverages on the day of the survey. This proportion increased to 50 percent among children 36 to 47.9 months of age, making sugar-sweetened beverage intake more prevalent than 100 percent fruit juice intake in this age group. Children 12 months of age and older who reportedly consumed sugar-sweetened beverages on the day of the survey, consumed approximately 100–110 calories from such products, said Story. Sugar-sweetened beverages contribute to 5 percent of total calories per capita among children 12 to 17.9 months of age, a proportion that increases to 10 percent among children 36 to 47.9 months of age. Among the different types of sugar-sweetened beverages, fruit-flavored drinks are the most commonly consumed type and contribute to the majority of sugar-sweetened beverage calories consumed among children 0 to 47.9 months of age.

Story touched on trends in beverage intake across FITS 2002, 2008, and 2016 data. Drawing a parallel with the evidence presented by Siega-Riz, Story showed that the prevalence of 100 percent fruit juice intake has decreased over time in all evaluated age groups. In contrast, the trends in the prevalence in sugar-sweetened beverage intake over time are mixed across the evaluated age groups. Some age groups appear to have decreased intake over time (e.g., children 21 to 24 month of age), while other age groups appear to have slightly increased intake (e.g., children 9 to 12 months of age).

Differences emerged when sugar-sweetened beverage intake was evaluated by race and ethnic groups. Intake was more common and, among consumers, contributed more calories per day among non-Hispanic black children 24 to 47.9 months of age than among non-Hispanic white and Hispanic children in the same age range. Story explained that these differences were primarily driven by more widespread fruit-flavored drink intake among non-Hispanic black children.

At the end her presentation, Story described potential future analyses of the FITS 2016 data and discussed what she perceived as evidence gaps. She suggested that opportunities exist to use FITS 2016 to explore beverage intake patterns by meal and snack occasion, by location (including different child care settings as compared to the home setting), and by income level. Speaking more broadly, Story thought that opportunities exist to better understand parent and caregiver attitudes and beliefs regarding beverages in the diets of young children, especially health beliefs about fruit-flavored drinks. Story also believes a need exists to better understand sugar-sweetened beverage intake in the context of overall dietary intake and diet quality, including as it relates to total energy intake and consumption of fruits, vegetables, and whole grains. She concluded her presentation by proposing that more data are needed on young children 48 months of age and older.

COST-EFFECTIVE STRATEGIES TO LIMIT SUGAR-SWEETENED BEVERAGES IN CHILDREN: WHAT CAN WE EXPECT?[3]

In his presentation, Gortmaker described select findings from the Childhood Obesity Intervention Cost-Effectiveness Study (CHOICES) (President and Fellows of Harvard College, 2015). CHOICES is a project that aims to estimate the cost-effectiveness and population health effect of obesity prevention programs and policies. Gortmaker's team has assessed nearly 50 obesity strategies and has searched for evidence of effect by performing systematic reviews on more than 130,000 peer-reviewed articles. Drawing

[3] This section summarizes information presented by Steven Gortmaker.

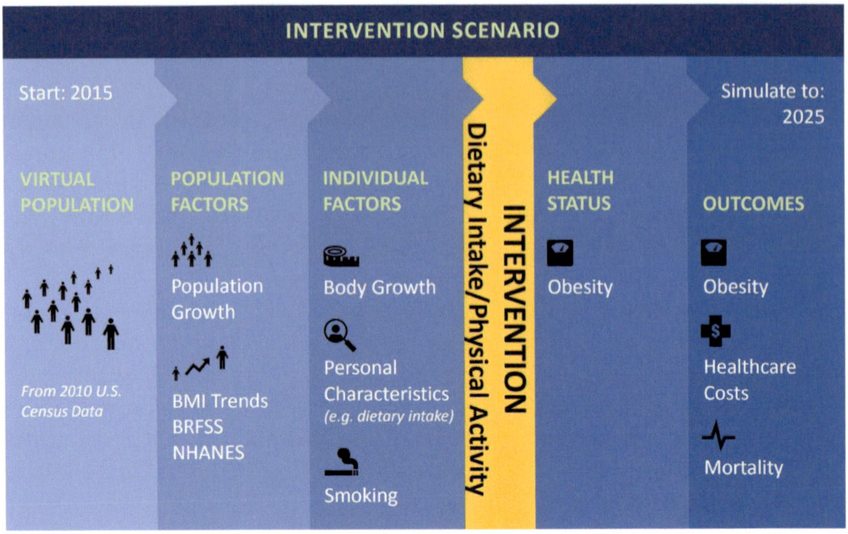

FIGURE 2-1 Approach to creating microsimulation models for dietary intake and physical activity intervention scenarios as part of the Childhood Obesity Intervention Cost Effectiveness Study (CHOICES).
NOTE: BMI = body mass index; BRFSS = Behavioral Risk Factor Surveillance System; NHANES = National Health and Nutrition Examination Study.
SOURCE: As presented by Steven Gortmaker, June 21, 2017.

on big data at the national, state, and local levels, Gortmaker's team has created microsimulation models to estimate the cost-effectiveness of an intervention over a 10-year period and to project how it would affect health outcomes such as obesity and mortality (Cradock et al., 2017; Dietz and Gortmaker, 2016; Gortmaker et al., 2015) (see Figure 2-1). The models require "estimates of reach, estimates of effect, and cost," he noted.

Through CHOICES, Gortmaker's team has evaluated strategies directly related to sugar-sweetened beverages, a category of beverages he defined as including "soda, sports drinks, fruit drinks and punches, [and] sweetened tea," but not including flavored milk or 100 percent fruit juice. Citing evidence from Wang et al. (2008), which showed that children 2 to 5 years of age consume the majority of calories from sugar-sweetened beverages at home, Gortmaker suggested that interventions likely to have the greatest effect on the intake among young children are those that affect the home setting.

The evidence to support the effect of changing sugar-sweetened beverage intake on body mass index and obesity in children is "quite strong," noted Gortmaker. An 18-month double-blind, randomized trial of sugar-free and sugar-sweetened beverages in Dutch children 4 to 11 years of age provides evidence that sugar-sweetened beverage intake affects relative weight (de Ruyter et al., 2012). Another analysis of the Dutch study data found that children with higher body mass indexes may not compensate as much as leaner children when the sugar-sweetened beverages are replaced with sugar-free beverages (Katan et al., 2016). In considering the applicability to U.S. children, Gortmaker observed that the higher body mass index group in the Dutch analyses was comparable to the average body mass index among children 6 to 11 years of age in the United States (Ogden et al., 2012). Accordingly, he thought the effect on body weight status may be underestimated for U.S. children. Evidence of the effect of changing sugar-sweetened beverage intake on body weight status in young children birth to 5 years of age is less robust. Gortmaker explained that fewer studies are conducted in this age range and that collecting accurate dietary intake data on young children is an issue because it is "pretty hard to know how much went in their mouth, how much went on the floor, [and] what did they really consume." Nevertheless, he suggested that the relationship documented in other age groups is likely to exist in younger children.

After providing the context of evidence of effect, Gortmaker described the published results from his group's microsimulation models for three interventions: sugar-sweetened beverage excise tax, Smart Snacks in Schools, and the Nutrition and Physical Activity Self-Assessment for Child Care (NAP SACC) (Gortmaker et al., 2015). Owing to differences in scale and expected reach, the interventions had various projected outcomes of cases of obesity prevented over a 10-year period and cost-effectiveness. Speaking broadly about the interventions his group has modeled, Gortmaker remarked that few result in cost savings.

The models indicate that a one-cent-per-ounce excise tax on sugar-sweetened beverages, if implemented across the United States, would have the greatest effect of the three interventions. The excise tax is projected to prevent nearly 580,000 cases of childhood obesity and to provide more than $30 in health care cost savings for every $1 invested, noted Gortmaker. He further explained that an increase in the price of sugar-sweetened beverages would lead to lower consumption, especially among population groups that have higher intake. As such, the sugar-sweetened beverage excise tax has the potential to reduce racial/ethnic and socioeconomic disparities in intake (Long et al., 2016). It could further improve health equity, observed Gortmaker, if the estimated $12.5 billion in revenue generated per year from the tax were to be invested in other preventative activities. He acknowledged that limited work is currently being done to evaluate the effect of existing sugar-sweetened beverage taxes on children, and he identified this as a research opportunity.

Smart Snacks in Schools is expected to have similar effects as the sugar-sweetened beverage excise tax, but to a lesser degree. The microsimulation model estimated that Smart Snacks in Schools would prevent approximately 345,000 cases of childhood obesity, and would result in a nearly $5 health care cost savings for every $1 invested, Gortmaker said.

NAP SACC is an intervention used to change the nutrition profile of food provided in the early care and educational setting. Gortmaker reported that because it would have a smaller reach than the sugar-sweetened excise tax and the Smart Snacks in Schools initiative, NAP SACC is projected to prevent far fewer cases of childhood obesity—approximately 38,000 cases. In contrast to the two other interventions, NAP SACC would not result in health care cost savings, but instead would only return $0.04 to $0.08 for every $1 invested, he continued. The NAP SACC microsimulation model offered additional findings of interest. Although it is likely to not have a large effect on obesity, the models indicated that replacing 100 percent fruit juice with water in a typical child care center with 30 children could save approximately $1,000 per year at that center, noted Gortmaker. He emphasized that sugar-sweetened beverage habits and practices start early in life, and that opportunities exist to make early care and educational settings healthier.

Gortmaker pointed out that when modeling the effects of interventions limiting 100 percent fruit juice consumption, changes in intake lead to changes in weight in adults (Mozaffarian et al., 2011). He explained that it is difficult to detect such a relationship in children because of the limitations of current data and because there are few longitudinal studies of young children. Emphasizing a point he made earlier in his presentation, Gortmaker thought that unreliable dietary intake data is one reason the relationship between change in 100 percent fruit juice intake and change in weight in children has been inconsistent in the literature. In presenting results from Ludwig et al. (2001), Gortmaker underscored the importance of analyses evaluating change in sugar-sweetened beverage intake with change in body mass index, rather than looking at baseline intake alone.

DRINKING WATER: WHAT DO WE NEED TO KNOW AND DO?[4]

Although limited in nature, evidence suggests that infants and toddlers are adequately hydrated, but are likely to be under-hydrated by the time they reach school age (Drewnowski et al., 2013; Grimes et al., 2017; Kant et al., 2010; Kenney et al., 2015b). Presenting evidence from recent NHANES analyses, Hecht noted that the majority of, but not all, children 6 months through 5 years of age reportedly consume water (Grimes et al.,

[4] This section summarizes information presented by Christina Hecht.

2017; Watowicz et al., 2015). Further emphasizing this point, she reported that an analysis using 2005–2010 NHANES data found that 83 percent of children 1 to 19 years of age consumed tap water, 10 percent consumed bottled water, and 7 percent reportedly consumed no water (Patel et al., 2013). Tap water consumption was less common among female, Hispanic, and black children and was twice as common among children with a college-educated parent (Patel et al., 2013). Hecht described tap water as economical, "a disparity reducer," and, when fluoridated, a contributor to oral health. Given that unhealthy beverage intake patterns start developing in early childhood, "We want to make plain water the normative beverage after age-appropriate amounts of milk in this age group," said Hecht. To establish water intake as a habit in young children, Hecht highlighted the importance of safety, access, and promotion.

Water Safety

Infant formula, which is typically prepared using tap water, is consumed by the majority of infants in the United States (Grimes et al., 2017; Miles and Siega-Riz, 2017). Hecht noted that 60 percent of infants 0 to 5 months of age are exclusively formula fed. The risk of exposure to lead in tap water is a concern in formula-fed infants because they can consume upwards of 4 cups of infant formula per day, which is more water in proportion to body weight than any other age group. Lead is particularly toxic to children younger than 7 years of age because they have greater gastrointestinal absorption and are more vulnerable to the neurotoxic effects, stated Hecht. She noted that other factors associated with formula feeding, such as socioeconomic status and zip code, also appear to be associated with an elevated risk of unsafe tap water (Edwards et al., 2009).

Hecht explained that there are two categories of water contamination. One category is contaminated source water that is not properly treated by the water utility. Approximately 5 percent of water utilities provide contaminated water to their customers, she noted. The other source of water contamination occurs after leaving the main line of the water utility. When service lines are made of lead or when lead is present in premise plumbing, lead can either leach or flake into the water and contaminate it (Triantafyllidou and Edwards, 2012).

Despite a lack of surveillance data, evidence drawn from media reports indicates that tap water contamination occurs throughout the United States (see Figure 2-2), suggesting that "existing regulations, guidelines, and systems do not always safeguard our water," said Hecht. She explained that there are locations particularly susceptible to unsafe water, including "areas subject to agricultural runoff, industrial pollution, mining or fracking activities, and rural and inner-city areas." Hecht reported that, to date,

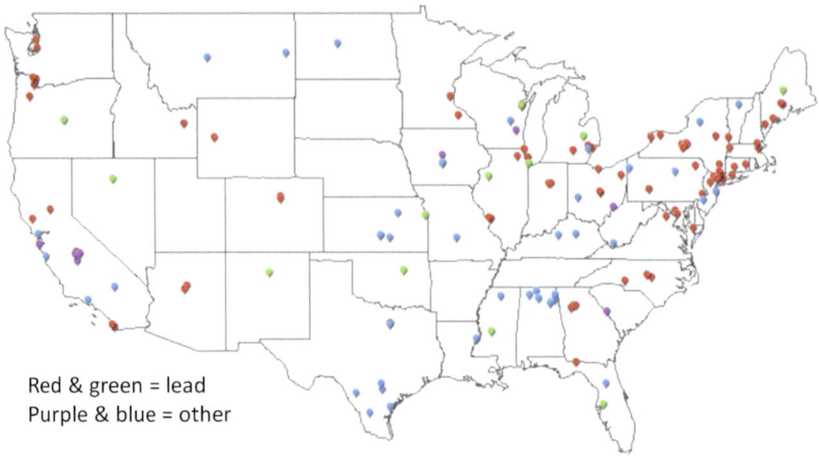

FIGURE 2-2 Media reports of tap water contamination since January 2015.
SOURCES: As presented by Christina Hecht, June 21, 2017. Copyright © 2017 The Regents of the University of California. Used by permission.

only 14 states and the District of Columbia have mandatory or voluntary testing of lead in school tap water, and each varies in its approach to testing. In New York State, which has mandatory testing, nearly 12 percent of taps had lead levels exceeding 15 parts per billion,[5] the action level set by the U.S. Environmental Protection Agency. Even fewer states have provisions regarding testing tap water in child care settings. Hecht recounted a conversation she had with a coordinator of the Rhode Island Department of Health program offering voluntary testing in Rhode Island child care centers. The coordinator indicated that participation in the program had been low because the child care centers feared the cost of remedying any issue found. As another example, Hecht noted that mandatory testing in the state of Washington is contingent on appropriated funding and, at the time of the workshop, funding had yet to be allocated.

Water Access and Consumption

When improved access to water is paired with education, water consumption is increased, explained Hecht, who used two studies to exemplify her point. A trial in German elementary schools by Muckelbauer et al. (2009) showed that increased access to water fountains and reusable

[5] Later in her presentation Hecht noted that the American Academy of Pediatrics recommends that school water fountains should have water lead concentrations that do not exceed one part per billion (Council on Environmental Health, 2016).

bottles, coupled with teacher-led education on water, increased students' daily water intake by 220 milliliters and reduced the risk of overweight in the intervention schools as compared to the control schools. Kenney et al. (2015a) reported that providing access to cups during school lunch and promoting water through posters increased the number of students who consumed water, increased the amount of water students consumed, and appeared to reduce the number of students who consumed sugar-sweetened beverages. Similar trials in the child care setting are lacking, observed Hecht.

Hecht stated, "Policy on water can be a key lever for access," noting that such policies exist in the federal child nutrition programs. Effective October 1, 2017, providers participating in the Child and Adult Care Food Program (CACFP) are required to make water available as well as to offer water with visual cues over the course of the day. Hecht highlighted that the new CACFP standards are well-aligned with recent recommendations made by the American Academy of Pediatrics and by an expert panel convened by the Robert Wood Johnson Foundation Healthy Eating Research program. She also noted that the update in policy affects not only CACFP providers (which includes one-half of all licensed child care providers), but also the licensed child care providers in the one-half of U.S. states that link licensure nutrition standards to CACFP regulations.

Water Promotion

Hecht emphasized the importance of drinking water promotion and education, together with improving access, as a key facilitator in boosting water consumption in preference to sugar-sweetened beverages, and she showed a variety of promotional materials aimed at the early years. Hecht concluded by outlining barriers to and opportunities for the role of drinking water access and promotion in an effort to eliminate sugar-sweetened beverage consumption in children 0 to 5 years of age. She suggested that barriers include gaps in the evidence base including the lack of definitive evidence that increased water consumption does not displace other healthy beverages and foods in the diet, although preliminary findings suggest it does not (Ritchie et al., 2012).

Hecht believes that misperceptions about water safety are a more substantial barrier than actual safety, but she noted that evidence gaps about safety do exist. She also emphasized the importance of modeling behaviors and that many parents and caregivers drink sugar-sweetened beverages themselves. Hecht recognized that parents and caregivers also receive a range of mixed messages regarding healthy beverages. To rectify this, she thought an opportunity exists to improve clarity for parents and caretakers on what beverages children should be drinking, how the beverages should be offered, and how much of the beverage should be provided. She also suggested that education is a necessary component of water promotion and could be enhanced by including strong language in the *2020–2025 Dietary Guidelines for Americans* and adding a symbol for water on the MyPlate graphic.

FACILITATED DISCUSSION WITH THE AUDIENCE

Following the presentations, Birch moderated a facilitated discussion between the audience and Siega-Riz, Story, Gortmaker, and Hecht. The sections below summarize topics that emerged during the conversation.

Data Quality and Evidence Gaps

Birch opened the facilitated discussion by asking the session speakers what data would be ideal to fill existing gaps. Story thought that there should be greater investment in improving dietary assessment methods. She acknowledged that groups are currently working on this issue, innovating through use of smartphones and use of pictures. Building on this point, Gortmaker noted that an opportunity exists, such as using phones to take pictures or videos, to "gather more precise estimates to validate all the recall methods." Bringing the conversation specifically back to beverages, Story believed that people were more aware of what kind and what size beverage they consume than how much they eat. Hecht wondered if packaged beverages were more readily recalled than tap water. Related to this topic, Hecht reiterated a point made during her presentation: more data on tap water quality is needed.

Noting that she was less concerned with the precision of dietary intake data than with the overall trend, Siega-Riz explained that understanding how beverage consumption tracks with weight in children is challenging, because data are largely cross-sectional. She identified the lack of longitudinal data on U.S. children from birth as a major gap in existing evidence. Siega-Riz further explained that sample sizes in NHANES for young children are relatively small, limiting the number and types of additional analyses or subgroup comparisons that can be performed. When an audience member proposed looking at sugar-sweetened beverage consumption by acculturation status, Siega-Riz noted that the NHANES sample would be too small, especially if also broken down by age group.

Testing of Drinking Water

Drawing from an audience member-submitted question, Birch asked Hecht to describe what has facilitated the passing of regulations for testing tap water in schools and child care facilities. Although she admitted to not knowing the background of what happened in every state, Hecht explained that in California "it was thanks to the work of a very strong network of drinking water advocates who work on all sorts of drinking water issues." Siega-Riz emphasized that the map that Hecht showed during her presentation (see Figure 2-2) was based on media reports, and as such most likely reflected a sizeable underestimation of contamination in the United States. Drawing attention to this, she suggested that mandatory testing would be needed to truly understand the scope of water safety issues nationwide.

Gortmaker remarked that funds are generally allocated for testing rather than remedying any issues found, although Hecht noted that the initiative in California has money for both testing and remediation. Siega-Riz proposed that some of the funds from the excise tax on sugar-sweetened beverages could be put toward resolving water contamination issues found through testing, creating what she perceived as "a win-win solution." Hecht agreed with Siega-Riz, but thought this approach could create equity issues, given where the sugar-sweetened beverage excise taxes have been approved at the city level.

100 Percent Fruit Juice

Birch posed a series of audience questions regarding 100 percent fruit juice. An audience member wanted to know about the dietary effects of 100 percent juice consumption. Siega-Riz explained that although 100 percent fruit juice does provide vitamin C, it does not provide fiber and some of the nutrients that are found in whole fruit. When asked if 100 percent juice leads to greater sugar-sweetened beverage intake, Siega-Riz repeated a finding from her presentation—100 percent fruit juice is one of the first complementary foods introduced to infants. Gortmaker added that the longitudinal study of Sonneville et al. (2015) found that early juice consumption predicts later sugar-sweetened beverage consumption.

Location of Exposure

An audience member wanted to know if non-Hispanic black children are being exposed to sugar-sweetened beverages at home or in the child care setting, a question Birch believed was related to the data presented earlier in the session indicating that this population group had greater sugar-sweetened beverage intake. Gortmaker replied that in low-income populations, sugar-sweetened beverages are more likely to be found in family-based child care settings rather than child care centers. Siega-Riz hypothesized that the differences emerging in the Hispanic population may be attributed, in part, to the changes in the food packages offered by the

Special Supplemental Nutrition Program for Women, Infants, and Children (WIC) that took effect during the period evaluated.

Framing and Tailoring the Message

Birch posed a question from an audience member who wanted to know if any culturally tailored interventions to decrease sugar-sweetened beverage intake in specific racial or ethnic groups or in rural communities have been successful. Hecht noted that, based on responses provided during a focus group, parents may respond better to electronic promotion and electronic messaging (e.g., via phones, use of videos) than materials in written form. Siega-Riz added that messages need to be tailored to the culture and to the specific source of the problem.

Birch also asked the session speakers about tactics to target older siblings, caregivers, gatekeepers, and parents, as "children of this age do not make the initial decision to try a [sugar-sweetened beverage]." Story stated that we have to re-educate and increase the knowledge about limiting the consumption of 100 percent fruit juice. She also said that the message needs to get out that fruit-flavored drinks often have minimal or no actual fruit in them. Siega-Riz noted that to educate parents, translating the portion size into something meaningful is key, and consideration needs to be given as to how to provide clear messages to all caretakers of the child, including parents, grandparents, babysitters, and child care providers. Hecht thought potential messengers may be WIC staff and oral health care providers. In thinking about displacing juice in the diet, Hecht offered an anecdote. The head of a large child care conglomerate told her that when a center tried to make the switch to less juice and more water, parents felt as though they were not getting their money's worth. Hecht suggested that a strategy to combat this negative perception would be to make it clear that the money is spent on something beneficial for the children, rather than focusing on the removal of the juice.

An audience member asked the session speakers about adding sugar labeling or warning labels to products and how that would affect promotion to parents in terms of what is in beverages. Gortmaker and Story both expressed their support of the additional information about added sugars to the product labels. They both thought that if the sugar-sweetened beverage taxation was based on the amount of sugar in beverages, this could lead to the industry responding by reformulating products to lower the amount of sugar. Gortmaker also noted that the recent challenges to the sugar-sweetened beverage excise taxes in the United States have helped to educate consumers about sugar-sweetened beverages.

3

Beverage Intake Guidelines Applicable to Young Children

The second session, moderated by Esa Davis, associate professor of medicine at the University of Pittsburgh, focused on prominent national-level guidelines that offer beverage intake guidance applicable to children 5 years of age and younger. In the first presentation, Rafael Pérez-Escamilla, professor of epidemiology and public health at the Yale School of Public Health, discussed the scientific report of the 2015 Dietary Guidelines Advisory Committee (DGAC) (HHS/USDA, 2015b). Next, Stephen Daniels, professor and chair of the Department of Pediatrics at the University of Colorado School of Medicine and chair of the American Academy of Pediatrics (AAP) Committee on Nutrition, discussed existing AAP guidelines for beverage intake. In addition to discussing the recommendations for beverage intake, both presentations also provided insight into the evidence informing the guidelines. Following Daniels's presentation, he and Pérez-Escamilla took part in a facilitated discussion, moderated by Davis.

SCIENTIFIC REPORT OF THE 2015 DIETARY GUIDELINES ADVISORY COMMITTEE[1]

The *Dietary Guidelines for Americans* (*DGA*) provides food-based recommendations for individuals 2 years of age and older, and have "an enormous impact on all food and nutrition policy in the country, especially at the federal level, with very strong permeation to the state, all the way

[1] This section summarizes information presented by Rafael Pérez-Escamilla.

down to the local level," stated Pérez-Escamilla. He noted that the *DGA* affects various sectors, including the food industry (e.g., product formulation, reformulation), nutrition education policies, and food assistance programs. The *DGA* is developed through what he described as a three-step process: (1) scientific report of the DGAC, (2) translation of the DGAC's report into policy, known as the *DGA*, and (3) design and dissemination of *DGA*-related products. Pérez-Escamilla, a member of the 2015 DGAC, focused his comments on the topics, recommendations, and implication statements made by the 2015 DGAC relevant to the workshop.

Intake of Added and Free Sugars in Relation to Chronic Disease

The 2015 DGAC approached the evidence by conducting original systematic reviews, reviewing existing expert reports, performing food pattern modeling, and commissioning data analyses. The 2015 DGAC defined sugar-sweetened beverages as "liquids that are sweetened with various forms of added sugars," which include, but are not limited to, soda, fruitades, and sports drinks, stated Pérez-Escamilla. The DGAC primarily found moderate to strong evidence of the detrimental health effects of sugar-sweetened foods and beverages and refined grains, which included links to obesity, type 2 diabetes, heart disease, and dental caries. Echoing sentiments expressed by Anna Maria Siega-Riz in the first session, Pérez-Escamilla cautioned that the evidence was predominantly from studies on adults, as very few studies have been conducted on cohorts of children. Based on dietary pattern models and the scientific evidence on chronic disease risk, the 2015 DGAC concluded that added sugars intake should make up less than 10 percent of total energy consumed in the diet. Pérez-Escamilla emphasized that "added sugars should be replaced in the diet by selecting healthier options rather than replacing them with low-calorie sweeteners." He added, "there was absolutely no reason for [the 2015 DGAC] to endorse the use of low-calorie sweeteners in children." The 2015 DGAC also found moderate evidence to suggest that free sugars intake below 10 percent of total energy intake was associated with fewer dental caries, a conclusion that aligns with a systematic review by the World Health Organization (WHO, 2015).

Dietary Patterns

Recognizing that each individual nutrient, food, and food group does not independently affect chronic disease risk, the 2015 DGAC elected to consider the total diet in the context of dietary patterns. Pérez-Escamilla explained that low intakes of vegetables, whole fruit, and whole grains have resulted in markedly inadequate intakes of fiber in the U.S. population, which has implications for recommendations regarding the contribution of

100 percent fruit juice toward fruit intake. Pérez-Escamilla indicated that available evidence suggested energy-dense, low-fiber dietary patterns with higher intakes of "sweets, refined grains, and processed meats, as well as sugar-sweetened beverages, whole milk, fried potatoes, certain fats and oils, and fast food increase the risk of obesity later in life."

Food pattern modeling revealed that "it is very difficult to achieve a healthful food pattern when added sugars in food and beverages are consumed above 10 percent [of total energy intake]," said Pérez-Escamilla. He described the 10 percent limit on added sugars as "lenient." The analysis suggested lower limits were needed to achieve the goals set by the U.S. Department of Agriculture (USDA) food patterns over the course of a lifetime, as represented by different calorie levels (see Table 3-1). Pérez-Escamilla noted that other national and international organizations have arrived at similar findings regarding limiting added sugars (i.e., American Academy of Pediatrics, American Diabetes Association, American Heart Association, Centers for Disease Control and Prevention, World Health Organization), and he suggested that scientific consensus across organizations has had an effect on U.S. food labeling policy.

In the American diet, 19 percent of total energy intake comes from beverages, with 35 percent of beverage energy coming from sugar-sweetened beverages. Beverages (excluding milk and 100 percent fruit juice) make up 47 percent of the added sugars in the U.S. diet, with 39 percent of added sugars coming from sugar-sweetened beverages. Accordingly, the 2015 DGAC stated, "Dramatically reducing the intake of sugar-sweetened beverages and limiting sweets and desserts would help lower intakes of the food component added sugars" (HHS/USDA, 2015b).

Evidence-Based Policies

Pérez-Escamilla explained that very few policies are specifically directed at children 5 years of age and younger. Given that a 5-year-old is on the cusp of school age, Pérez-Escamilla mentioned that there is strong evidence for implementing school policies for nutrition standards to improve the availability, accessibility, and consumption of healthy foods and beverages sold outside the school meal programs. Reducing or eliminating unhealthy foods and beverages can help improve purchasing behavior and higher-quality dietary intake by children while at school, continued Pérez-Escamilla. From an implementation standpoint, he emphasized the role of schools and early child care and education settings. The 2015 DGAC recommended policies and programs in these settings be designed not only to limit unhealthy food and sugar-sweetened beverages and increase access to water, but also to support providers and teachers so sound nutrition education and physical activity is incorporated into the curriculum.

TABLE 3-1 Added Sugars Available in the U.S. Department of Agriculture Food Patterns (Healthy U.S.-Style, Healthy Mediterranean-Style, and Healthy Vegetarian Patterns) (in calories, teaspoons, and percent of total calories per day)

Calorie Level	1,000	1,200	1,400	1,600	1,800
	Empty calorie limits available for **added sugars** (assuming 45% empty calories from added sugars and 55% from solid fat)				
Healthy U.S.-Style	68	50	50	54	77
Healthy Mediterranean-Style	63	50	50	81	72
Healthy Vegetarian	77	77	81	81	81
Average	69	59	60	72	77
Average (teaspoons)	4.3	3.7	3.8	4.5	4.8
Healthy U.S.-Style	7%	4%	4%	3%	4%
Healthy Mediterranean-Style	6%	4%	4%	5%	4%
Healthy Vegetarian	8%	6%	6%	5%	5%
Average	7%	5%	4%	5%	4%

SOURCES: As presented by Rafael Pérez-Escamilla, June 21, 2017; HHS/USDA, 2015b.

The 2015 DGAC also highlighted the role of federal food assistance programs, recommending that programs be leveraged to support the purchase of healthier options, including foods and beverages low in added sugars. Pérez-Escamilla observed that the Special Supplemental Nutrition Program for Women, Infants, and Children (WIC) may be and can continue playing a role in the decline of not only sugar-sweetened beverages, but also 100 percent fruit juice consumption through revisions to the food packages offered by the program.

To help consumers make informed decisions, the 2015 DGAC specifically recommended that the Nutrition Facts label include added sugars, listed in grams and teaspoons, reported Pérez-Escamilla. He also noted that taxes are another factor that affects consumer decisions. While initially perceived as controversial when recommended by the 2015 DGAC, Pérez-Escamilla explained that sugar-sweetened beverage taxes, particularly the

2,000	2,200	2,400	2,600	2,800	3,000	3,200
122	126	158	171	180	212	275
117	126	135	149	158	194	257
131	131	158	158	158	185	234
123	128	150	159	165	197	255
7.7	8.0	9.4	9.9	10.3	12.3	15.9
6%	6%	7%	7%	6%	7%	9%
6%	6%	6%	6%	6%	6%	8%
7%	6%	7%	6%	6%	6%	7%
6%	6%	6%	6%	6%	7%	8%

tax implemented in Mexico, are effective policies for affecting intake and generating revenue.

Pérez-Escamilla noted that a disproportionate amount of marketing money is spent to promote unhealthy foods to children ($1.7 billion in 2009), as compared to healthy products ($80 million in 2009). Stating that racial disparities in marketing practices exist, he pointed out that 80 percent of foods and drinks advertised to children on Spanish television are unhealthy, and black children see more than twice as many television advertisements for sugar-sweetened beverages than their white counterparts. Websites and social media are also being used to promote food and beverages, particularly to children, Pérez-Escamilla remarked. The 2015 DGAC recommended that policies be implemented that limit exposure and marketing of foods and beverages high in added sugars and sodium to all age groups, particularly children and adolescents, specified Pérez-Escamilla.

Interface with Other Guidelines

Pérez-Escamilla concluded his presentation by noting that the Robert Wood Johnson Foundation's Healthy Eating Research (HER) program had recently put forth healthy beverage recommendations for water, milk, and juice intake of children 2 to 4 years of age and 5 to 10 years of age, which were consistent with the 2010 *DGA*. Pérez-Escamilla explained that the recommendations offer a strong message regarding juice, and that children do not have to consume juice if they prefer whole fruit instead.

AMERICAN ACADEMY OF PEDIATRICS (AAP) GUIDELINES[2]

One of the major areas of focus for AAP is providing nutrition guidance for children and adolescents. Daniels explained that AAP develops and publishes several types of reports and statements that provide various depths of analyses of the evidence:

- Clinical practice guidelines represent the highest level of evidence review, including a comprehensive review of literature and data analyses.
- Policy statements are based on a review of literature and describe and/or drive AAP's stance on a particular child health care and policy issue. They are considered "living documents" and are reviewed at least every 3 years, at which time the statement is "reaffirmed, revised, or retired," depending on the evidence that has emerged in the meantime.
- Clinical reports, also a type of policy document, aim to help the pediatrician make the best practice decisions based on current evidence.
- Technical reports focus on issues underpinning either clinical decision making or other types of issues related to pediatrics.

Daniels also acknowledged two major AAP publications that provide nutrition guidance for children and adolescents—*Nutrition: What Every Parent Needs to Know* (AAP, 2011) and *Pediatric Nutrition* (AAP Committee on Nutrition, 2013). Both are in the process of being revised.

According to Daniels, AAP has not formally defined sugar-sweetened beverages and, at this time, does not have a specific statement on beverage intake or sugar-sweetened beverage intake among children 0 to 5 years of age. He explained that AAP is currently developing a policy statement with the American Heart Association on the health effects of added sugars. AAP

[2] This section summarizes information presented by Stephen Daniels.

guidance, however, does note that a number of sugar-sweetened products (i.e., sports drinks, soft drinks, and energy drinks) are not appropriate beverages for young children.

AAP offers general feeding guidance for children younger than 5 years of age. During the first year of life (birth to 12 months of age), AAP recommends exclusive breastfeeding for approximately 6 months and continued breastfeeding throughout the first year of life, even after the introduction of iron- and zinc-rich complementary foods. Infant formula is the only acceptable substitute for breastmilk, noted Daniels, adding that cow's milk should not be provided to infants in the first year of life. He also highlighted a recent AAP policy statement recommending that 100 percent fruit juice not be given in the first year of life (Heyman and Abrams, 2017), a revision of a previous recommendation that 100 percent fruit juice could be offered to infants beginning at 6 months of age.

For the second year of life (12 to 24 months of age), AAP recommends that breastfeeding can continue and cow's milk can be introduced. Daniels noted that cow's milk should be the primary beverage for young children, starting at 1 year of age. He also explained that whole fruit is preferred, but that AAP guidance allows for 100 percent fruit juice to be offered to children 12 months of age and older. Accompanying this guidance is an emphasis on portion size—no more than 4 ounces of 100 percent fruit juice per day for children 1 to 3 years of age. To avoid risk of dental caries, 100 percent fruit juice should not be given in a bottle or at bedtime, stated Daniels. He added that calorie-dense and nutrient-poor foods and beverages should be avoided.

For children 2 to 5 years of age, Daniels said that AAP guidance places an emphasis on low-fat milk. He also specified that 100 percent fruit juice can help children meet their fruit intake goals, but only with appropriate portion size. For this age range, AAP recommends no more than 4 ounces of 100 percent juice per day for children 1 to 3 years of age and no more than 6 ounces per day for children 4 to 6 years of age.

Sugar-sweetened beverages are one of the top contributors to total energy intake for children, stated Daniels. He added that soft drinks are a main source of added sugars intake for young children and have been shown to displace milk in the diet. To encourage and sustain milk consumption and achieve nutrition goals for vitamin D and calcium, AAP recognizes that flavored milk can be part of a healthy diet. Daniels noted there is evidence to suggest that flavored milk can increase milk intake among children.

Pediatricians play an important role in monitoring growth, development, and changes in body mass index percentiles, which are used to evaluate whether dietary intake is adequate and to assess a child's progression toward obesity. Daniels thought that pediatricians should be tuned into cultural preferences to guide families toward the healthiest possible diet and suggested that health promotion efforts should aim to remove sugar-sweetened beverages from children's diets. He also believed that pediatricians should be asking parents about how they expose their children to media and help families develop a plan around media use. Outlining current media use recommendations, Daniels explained that pediatricians should discourage screen media for children 18 to 24 months of age, other than interactive applications, and, if media are to be introduced, high-quality programming and apps should be used. Children 2 years of age and older should be exposed to less than 1 hour per day of high-quality programing, with no screens during meals or 1 hour before bedtime, he continued. A family approach to sharing media should be used, noted Daniels.

To conclude his presentation, Daniels said that AAP is supportive of efforts to incentivize healthier eating and strongly supports WIC, the Supplemental Nutrition Assistance Program (SNAP), the school meal program, and policies that ultimately improve the diets of children. He stated, however, that AAP has not supported efforts to remove 100 percent fruit juice from WIC packages or efforts to disallow certain foods and beverages, including sugar-sweetened beverages, from the SNAP program.

FACILITATED DISCUSSION WITH THE AUDIENCE

To open the facilitated discussion, Davis asked Pérez-Escamilla and Daniels to discuss the strengths and limitations of different expert groups releasing guidelines on similar topics. Daniels noted that applying evidence is a challenging process that takes time, effort, and resources. He said that different groups may not arrive at the same conclusions because "there are major gaps in the evidence that require interpretation and, sometimes, insertion of expert opinion." Daniels also indicated that evidence-based guidelines are not always implemented, and suggested that more work needs to be done to understand how to enhance uptake. In describing how the DGAC scientific report is translated to the *DGA*, Pérez-Escamilla discussed the need for the process by which policies are created to be transparent and evidence based. He offered his experience with the HER responsive parenting infant and young toddler feeding guidelines as an example of how the committee involved in the review of the evidence had input on the translation of the evidence.

An audience member noted that the National School Lunch and School Breakfast Programs allow for up to 50 percent of fruit requirements to be satisfied by 100 percent juice, and asked if the regulations should be changed to only allow whole fruit. Daniels acknowledged that 100 percent fruit juice is not identical to whole fruit in terms of nutrition (e.g., fiber). However, he was not supportive of completely eliminating 100 percent fruit juice, given its portability and shelf stability. Instead, Daniels emphasized the role of the overall dietary pattern and how 100 percent fruit juice fits into the context of the total diet. Pérez-Escamilla suggested taking a life-course approach to developing preferences for unsweetened foods and beverages so that sugar-sweetened beverages, and perhaps even fruit juice, are not considered normative beverages for young children.

Davis posed a question from an audience member who asked about ways to restrict sugar-sweetened beverage purchases with SNAP benefits. Pérez-Escamilla explained that a few years ago he was part of an advisory panel asked to provide advice on whether USDA should administer SNAP more like WIC benefits (i.e., funds designated for the purchase of specific foods) or whether additional funds or incentives should be used to promote fruit and vegetable purchases. He noted there is opposition to imposing restrictions, particularly among civil society organizations working in very low-income communities. These organizations felt such limitations would target low-income communities and disallow choice. The advisory panel ultimately recommended launching the USDA Healthy Incentives Pilot to provide financial incentives for the purchase of fresh fruits and vegetables using SNAP benefits. Pérez-Escamilla also offered the idea of changing the definition of what qualifies as "food" so that sugar-sweetened beverages are no longer considered eligible. Daniels suggested leveraging SNAP Education to promote healthier food choices.

To conclude the facilitated discussion, Davis posed a series of audience questions related to milk. The first question asked whether the recommended alternative to sugar-sweetened beverages should be milk rather than water. Daniels repeated that, from AAP's perspective, there is a hierarchy of beverages for children with milk as the primary beverage, followed by water. The second question challenged AAP's position on flavored milk for young children, and suggested that unflavored whole milk should be recommended instead. Repeating a point made during his presentation, Daniels noted that when flavored milk is removed as an option, children who consumed flavored milk tended not to switch to unflavored milk. The final question Davis posed related to the sugar content in infant formulas. Daniels explained that both infant formula and breastmilk contain sugar. He said that infant formulas are designed to be compositionally close to breastmilk, and do not have the protein loads and other components of cow's milk that promote iron deficiency in infants. This compositional difference underlies the recommendation that cow's milk not be given to children younger than 1 year of age, stated Daniels. Pérez-Escamilla noted that emerging evidence suggests that one of the drivers behind the obesity risk difference between formula-fed and breastfed infants may be higher protein intake among formula-fed infants. Daniels suggested the obesity risk differences could also be caused by differences in hunger and satiety cues and mother–infant interactions.

4

Opportunities and Challenges to Influence Beverage Consumption in Young Children: An Exploration of Federal, State, and Local Policies and Programs

Christina Economos, professor and the New Balance Chair in childhood nutrition at the Friedman School of Nutrition Science and Policy and Medical School at Tufts University and co-founder and director of ChildObesity180, moderated the third session of the workshop. This session offered an overview of policies, programs, and practices at the federal, state, and local levels that affect beverage consumption in large segments of the population, particularly children 0 to 5 years of age. The session also sought to provide insight into the scope of the policies, programs, and regulations, including consideration of the population groups who are and who are not affected or served.

The first speaker, Sara Bleich, professor of public health policy at the Harvard T.H. Chan School of Public Health, described beverage-related regulations and policies in federal nutrition programs that serve young children. Next, Heidi Blanck, chief of the Obesity Prevention and Control Branch at the Centers for Disease Control and Prevention (CDC) in the Division of Nutrition, Physical Activity, and Obesity (DNPAO),[1] discussed the state and local public health opportunities to support healthy beverage intake. Natasha Frost, senior staff attorney at the Public Health Law Center, then spoke about state-level policies in child care settings. In the final presentation of the session, Kim Kessler, assistant commissioner for the Bureau of Chronic Disease Prevention and Tobacco Control at the New York City Department of Health and Mental Hygiene (NYC DOHMH),

[1] DNPAO is housed within the National Center for Chronic Disease Prevention and Health Promotion at CDC.

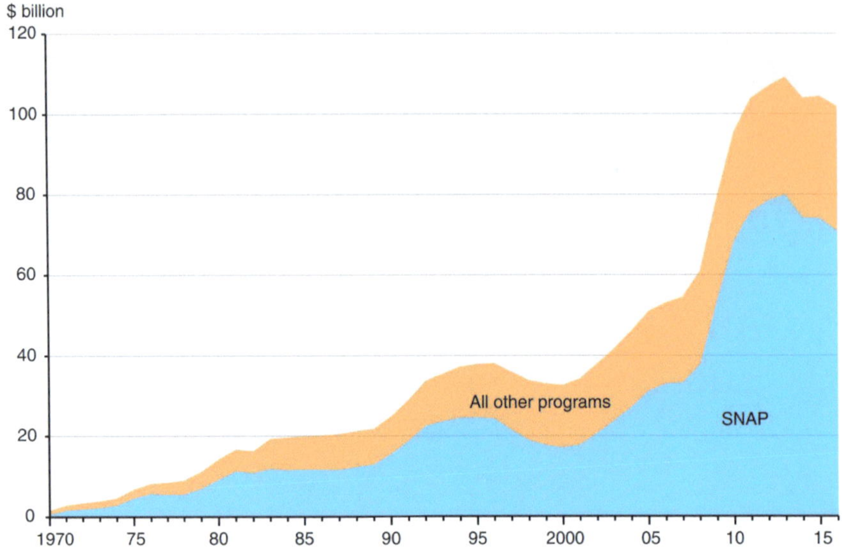

FIGURE 4-1 USDA expenditures for food assistance programs, fiscal years 1970 through 2016.
NOTE: SNAP = Supplemental Nutrition Assistance Program.
SOURCES: As presented by Sara Bleich, June 21, 2017; Oliveira, 2017.

provided a local perspective of New York City's strategies to reduce sugar-sweetened beverage consumption. A facilitated discussion with the audience, moderated by Economos, followed the presentations.

REGULATIONS AND POLICIES FOR BEVERAGES IN FEDERAL NUTRITION PROGRAMS[2]

The U.S. Department of Agriculture (USDA) administers 15 food and nutrition assistance programs that vary in cost and size, noted Bleich, as she provided context for her remarks. Expenditures for the programs, which exceeded $101 billion in the 2016 fiscal year, have markedly increased since 1970 (see Figure 4-1). Comprising 96 percent of the USDA food and nutrition assistance program spending, the five largest programs in descending size are the Supplemental Nutrition Assistance Program (SNAP); the National School Lunch Program; the Special Supplemental Nutrition Program for Women, Infants, and Children (WIC); the School Breakfast Program;

[2] This section summarizes information presented by Sara Bleich.

and the Child and Adult Care Food Program (CACFP). SNAP is by far the largest of the programs, serving approximately 44 million people per month and costing $70.8 billion in the 2016 fiscal year. Bleich pointed out that approximately one in four Americans make use of at least one of the federal food and nutrition assistance programs each year.

Children in the age range of birth to 5 years are served by seven of USDA's food and nutrition assistance programs. These include the five largest programs, along with the Summer Food Service Program and the Special Milk Program. Bleich provided an overview of select eligibility requirements and demographic characteristics of program participants. She showed that most of these programs have a requirement for participants to have an income equal to or less than 130 percent of the federal poverty level, but noted that WIC uses a higher income criterion of 185 percent or less than the federal poverty level. As compared to the national average, a larger proportion of participants in the programs are black. Highlighting the difference in participation levels in the School Breakfast Program (14.5 million children) as compared to the National School Lunch Program (30.3 million children), Bleich thought there was an opportunity to further leverage the breakfast program to expose more children to healthier options. She also indicated that participation levels vary by state, which she believed created opportunities to enhance enrollment of eligible children. Her assessment of the characteristics of children participating in the programs led Bleich to observe that, apart from statistics on participation levels, comparable data across the programs is challenging to find because information is often siloed in program-specific reports. The lack of uniformed indicators makes it difficult to readily identify data gaps and opportunities, expressed Bleich.

Bleich cited the 2009 update to WIC food packages and the 2010 Healthy, Hunger-Free Kids Act as two examples of recent changes that created better alignment between program policies and the *Dietary Guidelines for Americans*. She described the federal policies on sugar-sweetened beverages in the nutrition assistance programs as "setting a floor" that often allows for innovation at the state and local levels. According to Bleich, the beverage policies across the seven nutrition programs are relatively similar (see Figure 4-2). SNAP, however, is the only one of the seven programs that allows sugar-sweetened beverages to be reimbursed. Two other programs—CACFP and the Summer Food Service Program—allow for sugar-sweetened beverages to be served, but do not reimburse for them, Bleich said. She also drew attention to the similarities between the programs' policies and regulations related to flavored milk and 100 percent juice.

Describing the available data as "imperfect," Bleich briefly outlined beverage purchase and consumption patterns among SNAP and WIC participants. A recent report found that SNAP households spend approximately 5 cents of every grocery dollar on soft drinks, compared to

	Beverage type			
Program	**Flavored Milk**	**100% Juice**	**Other Sugar-Sweetened Drinks**	**Notes**
SNAP	✓	✓	✓	Must be non-alcoholic
WIC	✓	✓	✗	Milk fat level depends on age
NSLP/ SBP	✓	✓	✗	Flavored milk can be 0 or 1% fat Sugary and caffeinated drinks cannot be sold during school
CACFP	A	✓	A	SSBs can be served, but not reimbursed; no juice for infants
SFSP	✓	✓	A	Milk can be any fat level Other SSBs can be served, but not reimbursed
SMP	✓	-	-	Milk can be fat-free or 1%

Key: ✗ = Not allowed ✓= Reimbursable
A = Available (but not reimbursable)

FIGURE 4-2 Summary of reimbursement and availability of sugar-sweetened beverages in federal nutrition programs applicable to children birth to 5 years of age.
NOTE: CACFP = Child and Adult Care Feeding Program; NSLP = National School Lunch Program; SBP = School Breakfast Program; SFSP = Summer Food Service Program; SMP = Special Milk Program; SNAP = Supplemental Nutrition Assistance Program; SSB = sugar-sweetened beverage; WIC = Special Supplemental Nutrition Program for Women, Infants, and Children.
SOURCE: As presented by Sara Bleich, June 21, 2017.

4 cents per grocery dollar among non-SNAP households (Garasky et al., 2016). Bleich described the evidence as mixed regarding whether SNAP participants consume more sugar-sweetened beverages than those who do not participate in the program. The analysis and interpretation of the consumption data comparing participants and non-participants is complicated by selection issues, as SNAP participants are not randomly selected, noted Bleich. She thought higher consumption among SNAP participants could be more a function of socioeconomic status than program participation. The 2009 revisions to the food packages offered by the WIC program reduced the maximum allowance of 100 percent juice. Findings from Andreyeva et al. (2013) indicate sugar-sweetened beverage purchases declined after the food package change, and do not appear to be compensated for by purchases of other juices and beverages with non-WIC funds. Given its link to weight status, Bleich thought the reduction in the provision of 100

percent juice in the WIC program may have a positive effect on obesity risk of participants.

To conclude her presentation, Bleich provided her ideas for possible areas for improvement. She suggested that a "thoughtful conversation" is needed to discuss the possibility of restricting the purchase of sugar-sweetened beverages with SNAP benefits, and she emphasized that empirical data are needed to understand the effects of such a restriction. Bleich also suggested removing flavored milk as a permissible option in the WIC program. Touching on points she made earlier in her presentation, Bleich thought that participation of children in federal nutrition programs can be enhanced and that opportunities exist to further innovate at the state and local level. She ended by proposing that consistent metrics beyond participation levels across the nutrition assistance programs are needed to understand progress, identify gaps, and find solutions.

STATE AND LOCAL PUBLIC HEALTH OPPORTUNITIES TO SUPPORT HEALTHY BEVERAGE INTAKE[3]

Early nutrition begins with a mother's decision to breastfeed, continues as an infant transitions to family foods, and is maintained by those who care for the child outside of the home (e.g., early care and education [ECE] settings, schools), stated Blanck. Accordingly, she framed her presentation around DNPAO's three priority nutrition strategies that align with this life course concept: getting a healthy start, growing up strong, and maintaining good nutrition.

Getting a Healthy Start

Breastfeeding has been a long-standing priority area for CDC. DNPAO's work on this topic has focused on enhancing hospital support for breastfeeding women, providing support for employed breastfeeding mothers, and creating community-level support to make breastfeeding a normative and socially supported behavior, especially among low-income and African American women.

Blanck explained that the Maternity Practices in the Infant Nutrition and Care Survey, conducted by CDC every 2 years, largely functions as a "census of hospitals on the maternity care practices that are occurring to support breastfeeding." Each hospital receives a report of its self-assessment, and each state and territory receives aggregate summaries. Support is then provided to help make the hospitals better aligned with

[3] This section summarizes information presented by Heidi Blanck.

Baby-Friendly practices.[4] In 2017, 21 percent of U.S. babies will be born in a Baby-Friendly hospital, an increase from 1 percent in 2005, noted Blanck. Every state, the District of Columbia, and Puerto Rico each have at least one Baby-Friendly hospital.

Growing Up Strong

Blanck highlighted the role of ECE settings in supporting healthy growth. She briefly touched on the *Caring for Our Children* guidelines for ECE settings (AAP et al., 2011), which contain 46 standards relevant to obesity prevention that "go across many areas of the caloric balance, including healthy foods and beverages, physical activity, screen time, and breastfeeding."

Blanck then presented the "Spectrum of Opportunity" comprised of 11 obesity prevention opportunities that can be employed by state and local ECE systems (see Figure 4-3). Recognizing that the ECE landscape is highly decentralized and variable, DNPAO recently assessed policy and system indicators in every state (CDC, 2016b), as they relate to 7 of the 11 components of CDC's Spectrum of Opportunity. Blanck provided findings for three of the components: Quality Rating and Improvement Systems (QRISs), professional development, and facility-level interventions.

QRISs exist in 39 states, 29 of which include standards related to obesity prevention. South Carolina, however, is the only state to include language related to beverages. Blanck explained that for a child care program to receive the highest or middle QRIS rating in South Carolina, "sugar-sweetened beverages shall not be served."

Online professional development opportunities for ECE providers were found in 42 states. Over the past several years, DNPAO has worked to improve ECE providers' access to low-cost and free training opportunities. One such example is an on-demand healthy beverage module, which as of April 2017, nearly 2,000 ECE providers have taken.

Discussing facility-level interventions, Blanck stated, "Forty-seven states do promote or provide interventions, curriculums, or programs that can support healthy beverages." Several of the states are promoting self-assessments in family home and child care centers, using such tools as:

- Nutrition and Physical Activity Self Assessment for Child Care (NAP SACC) (UNC at Chapel Hill, 2017);

[4] Hospitals and birthing centers are accredited as *Baby-Friendly* if they meet specific guidelines and evaluation criteria related to infant feeding and mother–baby bonding practices, care, and support (Baby-Friendly USA, Inc., 2012).

- Let's Move! Child Care Advanced Checklist Quiz (Nemours Foundation, 2017); and
- Contra Costa Self-Assessment Questionnaire (Contra Costa Child Care Council, 2017).

Blanck also highlighted that DNPAO provides seed funding to ECE settings—18 states receive funding for nutrition-related projects, and ECE settings in all 50 states and the District of Columbia receive funding for physical activity initiatives. In conjunction with the Nemours Foundation, DNPAO has established an ECE learning collaborative to help support planning, development, and implementation of improvements.

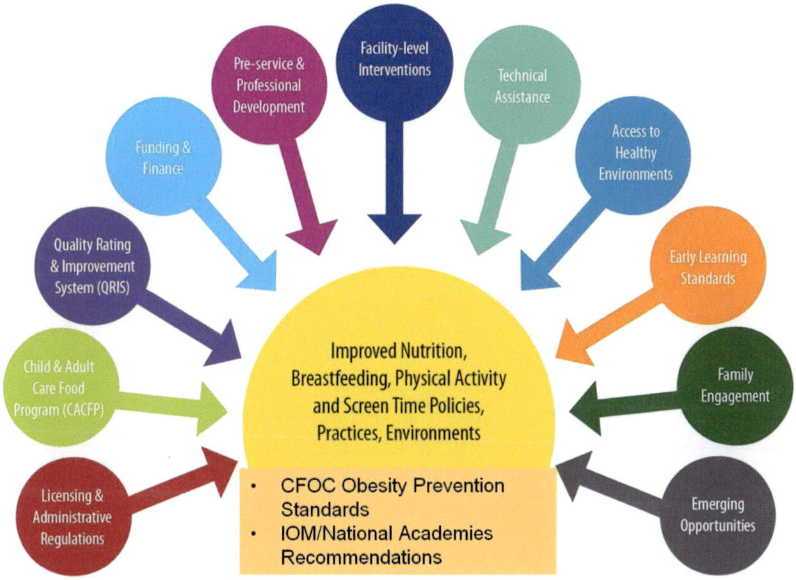
Facility-level Interventions
Pre-service & Professional Development
Technical Assistance
Funding & Finance
Access to Healthy Environments
Quality Rating & Improvement System (QRIS)
Early Learning Standards
Child & Adult Care Food Program (CACFP)
Family Engagement
Licensing & Administrative Regulations
Emerging Opportunities
Improved Nutrition, Breastfeeding, Physical Activity and Screen Time Policies, Practices, Environments
• CFOC Obesity Prevention Standards
• IOM/National Academies Recommendations

FIGURE 4-3 Spectrum of opportunities for obesity prevention in early care and education settings.
NOTES: CFOC = Caring for Our Children; IOM = Institute of Medicine; National Academies = National Academies of Sciences, Engineering, and Medicine. This figure was modified from what the speaker presented to reflect that as of March 15, 2016, the National Academies of Sciences, Engineering, and Medicine continue the consensus studies and convening activities previously undertaken by the Institute of Medicine.
SOURCES: As presented by Heidi Blanck, June 21, 2017; CDC, n.d. (modified).

Maintaining Good Nutrition

CDC has released a number of toolkits, guidelines, and frameworks to improve various nutrition environments, explained Blanck. One toolkit, for example, provides guidance on increasing drinking water access in ECE settings (CDC, 2014a). Other resources pertain to the school setting, including addressing competitive foods, promoting healthier options, and increasing drinking water access (CDC, 2011, 2014b, 2016a). More broadly, CDC offers food service guidelines for federal facilities, which Blanck noted can be adapted for "hospitals, parks and recreation venues, worksites, and community vending" (Food Service Guidelines Federal Workgroup, 2017). She also highlighted the Community Health Media Center, which serves as a centralized resource of materials used in CDC's local community projects that other communities can use (CDC, 2013). The education component of SNAP (SNAP-Ed), noted Blanck, also has a toolkit and evaluation framework of obesity strategies, made available by the National Collaborative on Childhood Obesity Research (NCCOR, 2016). Finally, she shared that the American Academy of Pediatrics offers health care providers Next Steps counseling materials, which include English and Spanish information and activity booklets on a variety of topics, including sugar-sweetened beverages (NICHCQ, 2013).

STATE-LEVEL POLICIES IN THE CHILD CARE SETTING[5]

Strategic thinking is needed to promote health equity through laws and policies, as "laws and policies have often had adverse effects on some of the most vulnerable people in our society," began Frost. She suggested that, with the majority of children 5 years of age and younger spending a substantial amount of time in non-parental care, ECE settings represent a key mechanism for early intervention. Frost explained that *ECE environments* is a broad term that encompasses a range of licensed and unlicensed settings in which child care is provided by someone other than a parent. Her remarks focused on two such environments: (1) child care centers, which are generally located in a facility with multiple staff caring for a greater number of children, and (2) home-based care, which generally consists of one primary caregiver providing care for a smaller number of children in the caregiver's residence.

Child care settings are primarily regulated at the state level, stated Frost. Every state has different funding streams, quality measures, licensing and administrative regulations, and definitions for what qualifies as a child care center or family child care home. These differences have led to

[5] This section summarizes information presented by Natasha Frost.

a highly decentralized and heterogeneous landscape across the nation and have made drawing conclusions about these settings challenging, observed Frost. State laws underpinning child care settings and ECE quality measures generally do not contain stipulations regarding sugar-sweetened beverages. When they exist, provisions regarding sugar-sweetened beverages in the child care setting are typically found in licensing regulations.

Together with collaborators at the Harvard T.H. Chan School of Public Health and the Johns Hopkins Bloomberg School of Public Health, Frost has explored licensing regulations related to healthy eating, active play, and screen time across the United States (Public Health Law Center, 2017). They have found that licensing in most states does not contain a stipulation regarding limiting sugar-sweetened beverages in child care centers or family child care homes (see Figure 4-4). Many states, however, do have nutrition standards that are linked to the CACFP standards, which currently permit sugar-sweetened beverages to be served but not reimbursed. There are states, such as Mississippi, that have created their own nutrition standards separate from CACFP. Frost noted that only a handful of states have licensing regulations regarding serving sizes of 100 percent fruit juice provided in child care settings. In contrast, the vast majority of states re-

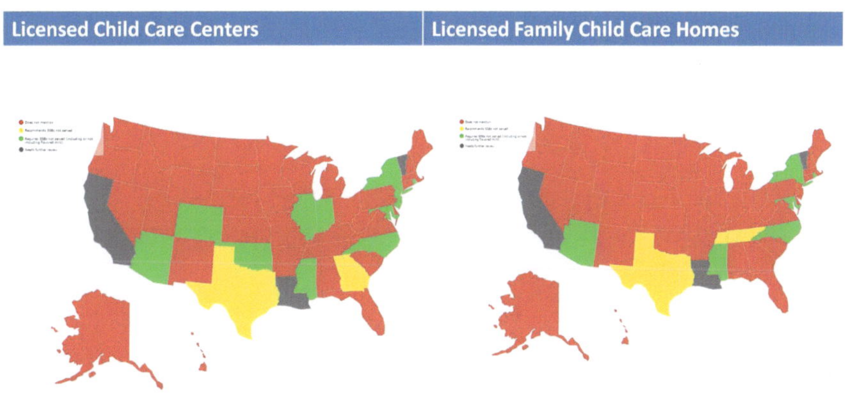

FIGURE 4-4 Child care licensing regulations with voluntary or required restrictions on sugar-sweetened beverages in licensed child care centers and licensed family child care homes.
NOTES: Red indicates limits on sugar-sweetened beverages are not mentioned in the state's child care licensing regulations. Yellow indicates the state's child care licensing regulations recommend that sugar-sweetened beverages not be served. Green indicates that the state's child care licensing regulations require that sugar-sweetened beverages not be served (may or may not include flavored milk). Gray indicates that further review of the state's child care licensing regulations is required.
SOURCES: As presented by Natasha Frost, June 21, 2017; Public Health Law Center, 2017.

quire that water be accessible throughout the day or in frequent intervals. "One of the things that we are finding about drinking water is that the implementation is really where it gets complicated," said Frost. She used Minnesota as an example to highlight possible unintended consequences. Frost explained that child care settings must provide either a water fountain or disposable, single-use cups, which has led to challenges and waste among facilities without a water fountain. She noted that the updates to the CACFP standards, scheduled to take effect in October 2017, also have a provision about water availability.

Frost then broadly discussed policy opportunities and considerations. She cited California's Healthy Beverage Statute as an interesting model for consideration, as stipulations regarding accessing drinking water and limiting sugar-sweetened beverages exist as a statute rather than in the licensing requirements. Given the variability that exists across states, Frost also emphasized the importance of local context when considering impact. Mississippi, for example, has nine licensed family child care homes, where Minnesota has 9,249 (Child Care Aware of America, 2017). In reflecting on her experience in Minnesota, Frost thought that opportunities exist for advocates and groups working on issues related to nutrition and ECEs to better coordinate with each other and to create a comprehensive strategy for state-level policies. She cautioned that action at the local level may not always be possible, as few states expressly permit local jurisdictions to implement their own nutrition standards. Frost concluded by suggesting additional consideration is needed to define quality in family child care homes, and additional research is needed to explore the role of such child care settings on the provision of sugar-sweetened beverages.

NEW YORK CITY'S STRATEGIES TO REDUCE SUGAR-SWEETENED BEVERAGE CONSUMPTION[6]

Health inequities exist in New York City, stated Kessler. She showed that neighborhoods with higher premature mortality rates track closely with neighborhoods that have higher concentrations of lower income and non-white households.[7] Furthermore, prevalence of obesity and diabe-

---

[6] This section summarizes information presented by Kim Kessler.

[7] Kessler presented maps showing the percentage of the non-white population, the percentage of the population below the federal poverty level, and premature age-adjusted death rates by New York City neighborhood. Sources of the data for the maps were cited as being from the New York City Department of Health and Mental Hygiene (NYC DOHMH) population estimates, matched from U.S. Census Bureau intercensal population estimates, 2010–2013, updated June 2014; American Community Survey, 2013, 3-year estimates, based on events occurring in 2014; population (based on zip code) defined as percent of non-Hispanic black and Hispanic residents, per 2010 Census; neighborhood poverty (based on community districts)

tes among black and Latino adults in New York City are approximately double that of their white counterparts. Adults' sugar-sweetened beverage consumption varies across the city, and there are higher levels of intake in many neighborhoods with higher rates of diabetes.[8] Kessler described the health outcome differences and reductions in life spans as "avoidable, unjust, and unfair." Accordingly, health equities are a priority area for NYC Health and are being addressed by considering the larger societal context and structural factors involved.

Kessler emphasized that sugar-sweetened beverages are widely available, generally inexpensive, and frequently served in large portion sizes. Such products are also heavily marketed to youth, low-income neighborhoods, and also communities of color, she continued. For example, a 2012 study found that 86 percent of food and non-alcoholic beverage advertisements in supermarkets and bodegas surveyed in the South Bronx neighborhood were for sugar-sweetened beverages. Kessler suggested that even when the marketing is not intended for young children, it can still have an effect by influencing family members who bring sugar-sweetened beverages into the home.

"We do our work with the awareness that even individuals with skills and the knowledge and the desire to make healthy choices will struggle to do so when the environment is working against them," stated Kessler. To that end, NYC Health seeks to "increase access to and awareness of healthy foods, and also decrease the availability and overconsumption of unhealthy foods."

One approach New York City is taking to achieve these goals is to promote healthy spaces for children. In 2006, the Board of Health updated the health codes for child care centers. The amendments included requiring appropriate serving sizes for 100 percent fruit juice (6 ounce limit), no longer permitting sugar-sweetened beverages to be served, and specifying that drinking water must be available and accessible. The health code was further revised in 2015, limiting 100 percent juice to children 2 years of age and older and reducing the maximum serving to 4 ounces per day. Similar requirements have been established for day camps.

New York City also seeks to transform its city and community environments. Food standards have been created that apply to the meals and snacks

---

defined as percent of residents with incomes below 100 percent of the federal poverty level, per American Community Survey 2011–2013; population (based on zip code) defined as percent of non-Hispanic black and Hispanic residents, per 2010 Census; and self-reported health—NYC DOHMH Community Health Survey, 2011–2013.

[8] Kessler presented maps showing the percentage of adults consuming one or more sugar-sweetened beverages per day and the percentage of adults with diabetes by New York City neighborhood. The source of data for the maps was cited as being from the NYC DOHMH Community Health Survey, 2011–2013.

purchased and served by city agencies and city-funded programs. The standards specify that beverages must be 25 calories or fewer per 8 ounces and that drinking water must be available at all meals. The standards also permit 100 percent juice within specific serving size specifications. Standards for vending machines in city spaces have also been established. Kessler explained the city's food standards have been adapted and used in other settings, including hospitals.

Kessler acknowledged that not all of the broad policy changes proposed by the city have been implemented. For example, a sugar-sweetened beverage excise tax was proposed in 2009 and 2010, but ultimately was not passed by the New York State legislature. In 2011, USDA denied a New York City petition to pilot and evaluate removing sugar-sweetened beverages as an allowable item for purchase with SNAP benefits. New York City also attempted to implement a portion cap on sugar-sweetened beverages, in an effort to "reset the defaults around portion size." Kessler explained that while these attempts did not result in policy, they did call attention to the issue.

New York City has also used educational campaigns to create awareness. Kessler noted that they have used hands-on nutrition education for the general public in various locations, such as ECEs and farmers markets, to serve low-income New Yorkers. To have a wider reach, New York City has also engaged in mass media marketing campaigns, which have included graphics (e.g., the "Pouring on the Pounds" campaign) and maps that use New York City landmarks to show how far one would need to walk to expend an equivalent number of calories in a sugar-sweetened beverage. Some of the campaigns have been youth focused (e.g., "Your kids could be drinking themselves sick.").

Kessler reported that there is evidence to suggest sugar-sweetened beverage consumption patterns are changing. Between 2007 and 2015, there has been a 34 percent decline of New York City adults' daily consumption of one or more sugar-sweetened beverages.[9] However, she stated that disparities still persist, as evidenced by racial/ethnic differences in daily sugar-sweetened beverage consumption.[10] Kessler reminded the audience that there is no silver bullet for improving diets in general and sugar-sweetened beverages specifically. Therefore, she emphasized the need for crosscutting

---

[9] Kessler presented adult daily sugar-sweetened beverage consumption data that were cited as being from the NYC DOHMH Community Health Survey 2015, and noted that the definition of sugar-sweetened beverages "includes soda and other sweetened drinks like iced tea, sports drinks, fruit punch, and other fruit-flavored drinks."

[10] Kessler presented adult daily sugar-sweetened beverage consumption data that were cited as being from the NYC DOHMH Community Health Survey 2007–2015. She also presented daily sugar-sweetened beverage consumption data cited as being from the Child Health Survey, 2009.

efforts. Kessler added that surveillance is critical for assessing programs and determining disparities that exist.

FACILITATED DISCUSSION WITH THE AUDIENCE

Economos began the discussion by asking the speakers, "To what extent are those who use the programs brought into the discussion for policy change?" Blanck replied that the Racial and Ethnic Approaches to Community Health program took a community-based participatory approach, a methodology she thought provides "the balance of understanding of what we as scientists think are evidence-based approaches and really the pragmatic feasibility of where community members think there are problems." Blanck also thought that perceptions of water safety need to be addressed through community input and awareness. She mentioned a study that found a higher distrust of U.S. tap water among Hispanic families, which was associated with higher sugar-sweetened beverage intake. In response to the question, Frost thought it is critical to engage child care providers to help think through implementation of proposed policies.

Economos posed several audience questions related to federal nutrition assistance programs. Speakers were asked their thoughts on whether CACFP should completely remove sugar-sweetened beverages as an option. Bleich thought that reducing exposure makes sense from a public health perspective, but the mechanics of implementation may be challenging. Blanck added that the lack of ECE surveillance data across the nation makes it difficult to understand whether sugar-sweetened beverages are actually being served or offered, and if so, whether it varies by CACFP status.

An audience member wanted to understand why the New York City waiver request for SNAP was denied by USDA. Kessler noted that USDA had indicated that it was because of the complexities of implementing such a waiver. Changing the universal product codes in the system is administratively burdensome, added Bleich. She also stated such a waiver would require having an evaluation plan in place to document the effect of the change. In considering an audience member's question about how to leverage federal nutrition programs to change the home environment, Bleich further elaborated on the concept of SNAP restrictions. She noted that the notion of SNAP restrictions has been around for quite some time, with strong opinions on both sides of the issue from advocates who care about helping low-income populations. In her opinion, Bleich thought that empirical data are needed to determine the effects of such a restriction and that a pilot trial would need to be authorized.

The speakers also discussed implementing policies and approaches for child care providers who are not located in centers, such as family, friends, and neighbors. Frost emphasized that approaches in such settings are locally and contextually specific. Funding and resource streams are also important considerations, she added. Blanck noted that one approach CDC has taken for such settings is the free or low-cost professional development modules. She also remarked that home environments have the ability to change much faster than other settings that require formal policies and rulemaking.

Responding to a question about the evaluation of the impact of communication materials, Kessler reported that there is evidence that obesity rates among some young children declined after the child care regulations took effect in New York City, particularly in high-risk neighborhoods. She noted that tracking outcomes related to communication products is much more challenging. Economos also posed a question from the audience about the Healthy Beverage Zone in the Bronx, and its potential as a national strategy. Kessler replied that the initiative is part of a collective impact model, in which NYC Health is one member of a coalition of organizations that are coming together to raise the health status of Bronx residents. She noted that as part of the initiative, organizations can opt into various types of healthy beverage-promoting activities, such as adopting an organization policy or promoting water.

5

Innovations and Challenges of Emerging Strategies

The fourth session of the workshop sought to explore novel policies, programs, and approaches to limiting sugar-sweetened beverages that have the potential to be implemented in other locations and scaled up. Henrietta Sandoval-Soland, food access director for the Community Outreach and Patient Empowerment (COPE) Program, described her organization's participation in the Notah Begay III (NB3) Water First! Learning Community and presented preliminary findings from a needs assessment conducted in the Navajo Nation. Marlene Schwartz, director of the Rudd Center for Food Policy and Obesity, then provided an overview of the policy, outreach, and media approach taken in the Howard County Unsweetened campaign. Following her presentation, she and Sandoval-Soland took part in a facilitated discussion with the audience, moderated by Tracy Fox, president of Food, Nutrition and Policy Consultants, LLC.

Next, a panel of speakers discussed the feasibility, challenges, and effects of local ordinances and regulations related to sugar-sweetened beverages. Each panelist gave a brief presentation to open the panel. Margo Wootan, director of nutrition policy at the Center for Science in the Public Interest, described the advocacy and policy approaches that have been used to make healthier items the default with restaurant children's meals. Lynn Silver, senior advisor at the Public Health Institute, discussed sugar-sweetened beverage excise taxes and presented key findings from an analysis of Berkeley, California. She also discussed the use of warning labels. Michelle Mello, professor of law at Stanford Law School and professor of health research and policy at Stanford University School of Medicine, highlighted select ordinances that have been subject to litigation. Following their prepared remarks, Wootan, Silver, and Mello took part in a panel discussion, moderated by Anna Maria Siega-Riz, which toward the end of the session expanded to a facilitated discussion with the audience.

COPE WATER FIRST INITIATIVE WITH THE NOTAH BEGAY III FOUNDATION[1]

The Navajo Nation is the largest tribe in the United States, with more than 170,000 members living in areas of Arizona, New Mexico, and Utah. Its residents, noted Sandoval-Soland, are disproportionately affected by poverty and unemployment as compared to national averages. To help create health equity and improve the well-being of Navajo Nation residents, the COPE Program, a nonprofit organization, focuses on issues related to access to healthy foods, chronic diseases (e.g., diabetes, cancer care), and educational outreach.

The COPE Program is currently undertaking a project as part of the NB3 Foundation's Water First! Learning Community. The Water First! Learning Community "seeks ways to increase consumption of safe drinking water or promote breastfeeding, as well as create healthy habits for children in their earliest years of life," Sandoval-Soland explained. The nine Water First! awardees will work during a grant period of 2.5 years to assess these issues to inform policy and system changes in their respective communities. Although each of the awardees has a different focus area,[2] opportunities exist throughout the award period for the grantees to convene and discuss progress, share ideas, and discuss strategies. One gathering hosted by the NB3 Foundation was the February 2017 Healthy Beverage Summit. The summit brought together not only the awardees, but also community members, organizations, and agencies to discuss reducing sugar-sweetened beverage consumption among Native American children in New Mexico and Arizona (Baca, 2017).

The Water First! Learning Community is aligned with the 2014 Dine Nation Act, which places a 2 percent tax on unhealthy foods in the Navajo

[1] This section summarizes information presented by Henrietta Sandoval-Soland.

[2] Sandoval-Soland briefly described the focus areas of the eight other awardees, as follows: (1) Five Sandoval Indian Pueblos are working with the Special Supplemental Nutrition Program for Women, Infants, and Children to promote breastfeeding; (2) Jemez Pueblo is focusing on policies and practices; (3) Mescalero Apache are focusing on youth-directed health education and activities; (4) Ramah Navajo School Board is focusing on policies and curriculum; (5) Santa Domingo Pueblo is using a community-based approach to promote drinking water and breastfeeding; (6) STAR School is focusing on clean water access and school-based education programs; (7) Tamaya Wellness Center is using education, marketing, and policy work to promote community attitudes and social norms; and (8) Zuni Pueblo Youth Enrichment Program is focused on hydration.

Nation, including sugar-sweetened beverages, Sandoval-Soland explained. The revenue from the tax is being invested back into the community to help support health and wellness projects such as vegetable gardens, greenhouses, farmer's markets, clean water, exercise equipment, and health classes, she stated.

Sandoval-Soland next discussed the design and progress of the COPE Program's Water First! project. She explained that the project's mission is to "increase access to safe drinking water among families with preschool children." Between October 2016 and June 2017, COPE conducted a needs assessment within the Navajo Nation. From July 2017 through September 2018, COPE will move on to what Sandoval-Soland described as the "implementation phase."

As part of their work during the first phase of the project, the COPE Program made a video that captures insight from a community elder regarding water and food (COPE Program, 2017). Sandoval-Soland emphasized the importance of this perspective, stating "We want to make sure that we are listening to the traditional knowledge of our elders."

To guide its needs assessment, the COPE Program developed a strategy map that contains four action areas (see Figure 5-1). Information was then

PERCEPTIONS	ASSETS & STRENGTHS
ACTION 1 - Agency Tour *How do our community members view children's health, water, SSB, Breastfeeding?*	ACTION 2 - Traditional Knowledge *What strengths in our community help to keep children healthy and well (healthy beverages)?*
ISSUES	**PARTNERS**
ACTION 3 - Meetings *What is happening now in our community with SSB, Water, Breastfeeding?*	ACTION 4 - Presentations *Who are and will be our partners in this work? What kinds of relationships do we need?*

FIGURE 5-1 Strategy map for the Community Outreach and Patient Empowerment (COPE) Program's need assessment.
NOTE: SSB = sugar-sweetened beverage.
SOURCE: As presented by Henrietta Sandoval-Soland, June 21, 2017.

gathered through a variety of ways, including surveys, interviews, focus groups, and community meetings. Sandoval-Soland noted that a central theme that emerged was that water is sacred and has importance beyond consumption, including being a part of ceremonial practices.

Sandoval-Soland shared some preliminary findings from the COPE Program's needs assessment, which consisted of 59 surveys collected across five Navajo Nation chapters. She highlighted a number of comments survey respondents provided regarding the influence of Navajo tradition involving food and beverages. Some of the respondents indicated that Navajo tradition affects how they regard or purchase foods and beverages (e.g., "It is a huge influence.") or that they would like to move more toward Navajo tradition (e.g., "I personally was not raised traditionally, but I'm in the process of learning traditional teachings."). Others indicated less of an influence (e.g., "I don't consciously think of my cultural values when buying and purchasing food or beverages; I usually buy what I know my family will consume"). Elements of tradition and belief emerged in feedback from respondents on the relationship between health and water (e.g., "Water is so important to Mother Earth." "I was told that water was always considered life." "Water is my clan."). Respondent comments revealed that family and kinship also influence food and beverage selections (e.g., "When food is prepared at home by the hands of my mother/sister/family members I know that it was made with love and reassurance. I feel safe eating it.").

The needs assessment provided insight into issues around drinking tap water, which included taste, perceived safety, and the color of the water. Sandoval-Soland explained that the findings from the needs assessment will inform the next phase of the project, helping to ensure that what is developed is traditionally and culturally relevant.

To conclude her presentation, Sandoval-Soland touched on the concept of incentives to promote change. Drawing on another COPE Program initiative as an example, she explained that her organization runs a food voucher program that promotes affordable access to fruits and vegetables and healthy eating in underserved communities. Sandoval-Soland thought a similar concept could be applied to improving water access.

HOWARD COUNTY UNSWEETENED: POLICY + OUTREACH + MEDIA = CHANGE[3]

To provide context for the Howard County Unsweetened campaign, Schwartz described the demographics of Howard County, Maryland. The county has a population of approximately 317,000 residents. The majority identify as non-Hispanic white (54 percent), with 18 percent of

[3] This section summarizes information presented by Marlene Schwartz.

residents identifying as black/African American, 18 percent identifying as non-Hispanic Asian, 7 percent identifying as Hispanic, and 4 percent identifying as other. More than one-quarter of county residents hold a professional degree. In 2015, Howard County had the fourth highest median household income in the United States. The proportion of students receiving free and reduced price lunch, which ranges from 4 to 40 percent in Howard County schools, suggests variability in income levels, noted Schwartz. She also added that the prevalence of overweight and obesity in the county (25 percent) is slightly below that of the state of Maryland (27 percent).

Howard County Unsweetened is a multidimensional, community-based initiative that seeks to improve the county's beverage landscape and reduce the consumption of sugar-sweetened beverages in particular. The campaign was led by the Horizon Foundation, which has a mission to improve the health of the county. "This was very much a community campaign that started in that community," noted Schwartz. Showing an image developed by the Horizon Foundation (see Figure 5-2), Schwartz called Howard County Unsweetened the "social ecological model in practice." Employing a multiyear, multicomponent strategy allowed the campaign to address different levels in various ways. During her presentation, Schwartz highlighted a handful of the project's components.

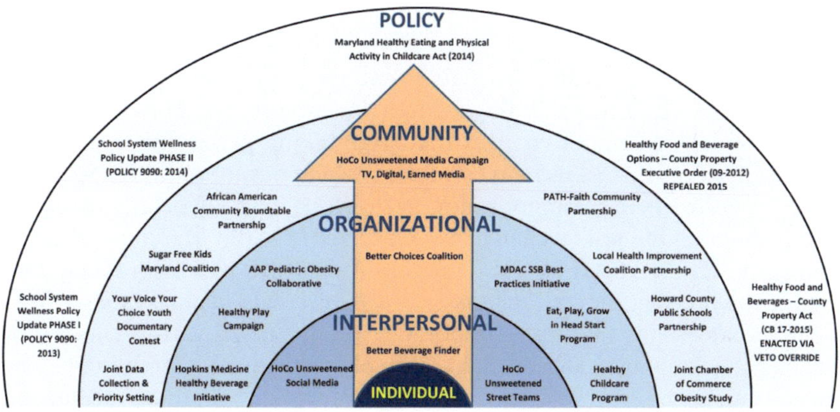

FIGURE 5-2 Social ecological model of the Howard County Unsweetened campaign.
NOTE: AAP = American Academy of Pediatrics; CB = Council Bill; HoCo = Howard County; MDAC = Maryland Dental Action Coalition; PATH = People Acting Together in Howard; SSB = sugar-sweetened beverage.
SOURCES: As presented by Marlene Schwartz, June 21, 2017. Printed with permission from the Horizon Foundation.

Schwartz described two of the individual- and family-level interventions of the campaign. She began with the Better Beverage Finder, which is a website that offers users alternatives to sugar-sweetened beverages as well as maps of where such products could be purchased in Howard County (Horizon Foundation, 2014). Those involved in conceptualizing the website thought it was necessary to not only focus on beverages to limit but also provide options for what could be consumed instead, noted Schwartz. Another component was a media campaign that included advertisements on local cable television, social and digital media buys, and direct mailings to county households. The advertisements primarily targeted mothers (e.g., "Want to make mornings easier? Try them unsweetened.") and specifically identified the beverages (e.g., "Sugary sports drinks can put children at risk.").

Howard County Unsweetened has several broader organizational- and community-level components. The Healthy Howard program, for example, was a project in which existing policies and practices within child care centers were evaluated. Providers were then helped to set goals to improve beverages, screen time, and breastfeeding support. Schwartz also described the update to the Howard County Public School System's wellness policy, a process that included an evaluation of the established and revised policies, along with public feedback. The Better Choices Coalition component of the campaign has community organizations, faith groups, and businesses agree to improve the vending and food options served at meetings and to educate visitors, members, and clients of the negative health effects of sugar-sweetened beverages. The Maryland chapter of the American Academy of Pediatrics formed a learning collaborative and developed a pamphlet physicians could use to educate their patients about sugar-sweetened beverages.

Schwartz explained that the changes that occurred in Howard County existed in the context of changes that were taking place within the state. The Sugar Free Kids Maryland Coalition, which has more than 250 members, generated media attention during this time as it advocated for state-level changes. One policy change that occurred was the Maryland Healthy Eating and Physical Activity in Childcare Act, which passed in 2014, and, among other things, limited sugar-sweetened beverages in child care settings.

Evaluation has played an important role in the Howard County Unsweetened campaign, shared Schwartz. She explained that initially, the messaging focused on "soda" and "sugary drinks." Evaluation data on beverage consumption by children led to the expansion of the messaging to include "fruit drinks" and "sports drinks," as these are more commonly consumed by children. She said that there is also messaging about limiting portion sizes of 100 percent juice, but to a lesser extent. Schwartz explained that the evaluation plan was developed before the campaign was implemented and consists of the following four components: assessing retail sales, conducting an annual survey of sixth grade students, coding child care and school policies, and performing health professional surveys.

In detailing the retail sales portion of the evaluation plan, Schwartz explained that 15 supermarkets in Howard County were matched with 17 supermarkets in a nearby state ("control state"). The stores were matched based on sales of soda, diet soda, sports drinks, fruit drinks, and 100 percent juice at baseline. The evaluation assessed changes in volume sales per product per week in Howard County as compared to changes in the control state. Schwartz reported that between 2012 and 2015, Howard County experienced a 20 percent decrease in volume of sugar-sweetened soda sold, while the sales in the control state remained unchanged. Sales of fruit-flavored beverages and 100 percent juice decreased more in Howard County than in the control state, while sports drinks remained unchanged in both locations. Diet soda sales did not differ between Howard County and the control state but decreased in both locations.

Schwartz also described findings from the annual survey of sixth grade students. She noted that the vast majority of students, approximately 97 percent, reported consuming water every day. "It is really not so much the regular soda as much as the fruit drinks that seem to be the most popular, followed by the sports drinks," Schwartz commented. Decreases in daily consumption of fruit drinks, flavored milk, sports drinks, flavored water and teas, regular sodas, energy drinks, and 100 percent juice were noted between the 2012 and 2016 surveys. When daily sugar-sweetened beverage consumption was assessed by racial and ethnic groups, some differences emerged. Black and Hispanic students reported higher average daily consumption rates than white and Asian students. Notably, all four groups of students reported lower rates of daily consumption in 2016 compared to 2012; the drops were significant for white, black, and Hispanic students. Despite these declines, black and Hispanic students continue to report higher rates of daily sugar-sweetened beverage consumption. Students were also asked about sugar-sweetened beverage availability in the home. Schwartz noted slight declines in fruit drinks and regular soda availability, but pointed out that these products are still in the majority of households.

To conclude her presentation, Schwartz highlighted key features of Howard County Unsweetened and discussed what she saw as future directions. She thought that one aspect that bolstered the success of the campaign was its origin within the community. She also emphasized the role of having an evaluation plan in place prior to implementation that is then used to guide the intervention. Schwartz acknowledged that while inroads are being made, sugar-sweetened beverages are still prevalent in the county and disparities exist. On the topic of disparities, she mentioned that the messages are beginning to be adapted to different population groups, such as including messages in Spanish.

FACILITATED DISCUSSION WITH THE AUDIENCE

After Schwartz's presentation, she and Sandoval-Soland took part in a facilitated discussion with the audience, moderated by Fox. Several of the audience questions posed by Fox asked the speakers to provide insight into how to implement an initiative, including considerations related to finding funding and persuading policy makers. Sandoval-Soland responded that community engagement and collaboration with local partners have been important. She said that one approach that has been helpful has been to use local champions to promote the cause and having the Navajo Nation tribal leadership onboard. Schwartz answered that in Howard County, there was the county government, a single school district for the county, and the Horizon Foundation, which had established connections and initiatives that could be leveraged. Schwartz emphasized that a focus on children also helps. "I think that politically, that was an easier sell. There is still quite a bit of work to do, and we see this as using all the tools in the toolbox to move forward," Schwartz commented. She added that funding was another important element, but thought funding should not be what dissuades a community from trying something. When questioned as to whether the Howard County Unsweetened campaign could be implemented in a less prosperous community, Schwartz countered by stating that children's health is a concern for any community.

Posing another audience member question, Fox asked the speakers to discuss possible opportunities to reduce children's sugar-sweetened beverage intake in the home environment. Schwartz stated that retail environments are affecting what people are bringing into their homes and it is for this reason that taxes, which affect people at the point of purchase, are so powerful. Schwartz also said that there are retail-based strategies, such as in-store placement and messaging, that may have influences on home purchases. Sandoval-Soland suggested that home visitation programs may offer opportunities to provide education about nutrition and health, and, specifically, reducing sugar-sweetened beverages.

LOCAL ORDINANCES AND REGULATIONS: FEASIBILITY, CHALLENGES, AND IMPACT

Healthy Defaults in Restaurant Meals for Children[4]

Wootan observed that parents often feel as though they are in control of their children's food choices, despite children frequently being in non-parental care (e.g., child care settings, school, after-school programs). Even

[4] This section summarizes information presented by Margo Wootan.

when parents are with their children, the food environment plays an important role in what foods children desire and are offered, she continued. Characterizing restaurants as "one particular place where children's diets get undermined," Wootan noted that approximately one-quarter of calories children consume are from away-from-home foods. When children eat out, they consume more sugar-sweetened beverages, calories, saturated fat, and sugars, and fewer fruits, vegetables, and whole grains as compared to when they eat at home, she explained.

The top food category marketed to children is restaurant food, stated Wootan. She indicated that the primary message children take away from fast-food advertisements is for them to go to the restaurant. The menu at the restaurant is another form of marketing and children's meals are marketed for young children. By bundling food items together for a reduced price, children's meals set defaults, which "set people's expectations for what they should do," she noted. Evidence suggests that changing the default options in children's meals to healthier options is highly accepted, and has an effect on the average calories in the children's meals ordered. She highlighted a finding from a study of Walt Disney World restaurants that found when the healthy beverage was the default in the children's menu, it was retained 66 percent of the time, despite soda being available for the same price (Peters et al., 2016).

Wootan discussed two approaches to change the defaults in children's menus: advocacy and public policy. Through partnerships and advocacy, restaurants have been encouraged to improve the dietary quality of their children's meals. Wootan described the progress toward making children's meals healthier as "modest." She shared, however, that through a variety of efforts (e.g., email, letter writing campaigns, Twitter campaigns, shareholders' actions) sugar-sweetened beverages have been removed from many children's menus. Approximately 75 percent of leading restaurant chains offered sugar-sweetened beverages on their children's menu in 2016 as compared to more than 90 percent offering such beverages in 2008, noted Wootan.

Wootan suggested that the slow pace of progress has led some communities and states to improve the nutritional quality of restaurant children's meals through public policy. The first two policies, passed in Santa Clara County and San Francisco, set nutritional standards for children's meals that come with a toy. Other policies have been passed in California (Santa Clara County and the cities of Davis, Perris, and Stockton) that change the default beverage in children's meals to healthier options. The options and standards for default beverages differ across the jurisdictions, but generally include unsweetened water and milk, with some allowing juice. Wootan suggested that the public policies aiming to improve the nutritional quality of children's meals have become less controversial and less contested over time.

Concluding her presentation, Wootan acknowledged that improving children's meals and removing sugar-sweetened beverages will not be a "magic bullet" and will not be the singular solution to the obesity epidemic. She argued, however, that restaurant food is heavily marketed and is a significant source of calories; making improvements to children's meals is a way to change social norms for children's food.

Taxation and Warning Labels on Sugar-Sweetened Beverages[5]

Silver began her remarks by noting that various approaches have been attempted by localities in the United States to limit sugar-sweetened beverages, including fiscal measures (e.g., taxation, Supplemental Nutrition Assistance Program restrictions), place-based regulations (e.g., child care, schools), product modifications (e.g., New York City portion caps, children's meal ordinances), retail environment changes, and marketing restrictions. In doing so, she highlighted that sugar-sweetened beverage excise taxes and warning labels are two strategies that exist within a broader context of strategies.

A sugar-sweetened beverage excise tax can influence health outcomes through two paths, Silver explained. First, the taxes will increase the price of the products, leading to decreased consumption and perhaps reformulation, which will reduce the risk of obesity and chronic disease and improve health. The second modality is through the revenue generated, which can be used for social investment and change, ultimately improving health and community well-being, Silver added.

In the past decade, approximately 60 sugar-sweetened beverage tax measures proposed in different localities in the United States have failed (Chriqui et al., 2013; Public Health Advocates, 2017; WCRF, 2015). Since 2014, however, such regulations have passed in nine jurisdictions (see Table 5-1). The existing sugar-sweetened beverage taxes vary in terms of the level of taxation, the products that are subject to the tax, and the uses of the revenue generated from the tax.

Evidence from the first year of a penny-per-ounce excise tax on sugar-sweetened beverages in Berkeley, California, has recently become available. Falbe et al. (2016) reported that sugar-sweetened beverage consumption decreased by 21 percent, and water consumption increased by 63 percent, in Berkeley's low-income neighborhoods 4 months after implementation of the tax relative to pre-tax consumption. Analyses using scanner data on over 15 million customer visits from two supermarket chains in Berkeley

[5] This section summarizes information presented by Lynn Silver.

TABLE 5-1 Sugar-Sweetened Beverage Taxes Approved in the United States, 2014–2017

Jurisdiction	Level of Tax	Products Covered	Use
San Francisco Oakland Berkeley Albany (California)	1¢ per ounce	SSBs only >25 cal/12 oz ≥2 cal/oz	General taxes with Advisory Committees or input guiding spending for health, obesity, and diabetes prevention
Navajo Nation	2% sales tax	Sweetened beverages and food of minimal nutritional value	Community Wellness Fund
Boulder (Colorado)	2¢ per ounce	SSBs only with ≥5 gms added sweetener per 12 oz	Dedicated to health promotion, wellness, and chronic disease prevention
Philadelphia (Pennsylvania)	1.5¢ per ounce	SSBs and artificially sweetened beverages	Pre-kindergarten education
Cook County (Illinois)	1¢ per ounce	SSBs and non-calorically sweetened beverages	General revenue, covering public safety and health needs
Seattle (Washington)	1.75¢	SSBs only ≥40 cal/12 oz	Childhood education and healthy food, water access, support to people with diabetes and obesity

NOTE: cal = calorie; gms = grams; oz = ounce; SSB = sugar-sweetened beverage.
SOURCE: As presented by Lynn Silver, June 21, 2017.

showed a 9.6 percent decline in sugar-sweetened beverage sales and a 3.5 percent increase in untaxed beverage sales during the first year of taxation (Silver and Ng et al., 2017). Silver noted that while sales of plain water and plain milk increased during the first year of taxation (15.6 and 0.6 percent, respectively), sales of diet soft drinks decreased (9 percent), despite being an untaxed beverage category. Scanner data suggest a 0.67 cent per ounce pass-through of the 1 cent per ounce tax on taxed beverages in Berkeley (Silver and Ng et al., 2017). Silver indicated there may have been a spill-over effect in nearby stores not in Berkeley, but stated that neighboring areas now have sugar-sweetened beverage taxes of their own.

Silver reported that there was "no increase in average grocery bill in these chains, nor greater decline in store revenue per transaction in Berkeley." The tax raised approximately $13 per person per year in Berkeley, which was fully used for health promotion activities. Silver acknowledged that there are no data on the effect of Berkeley's sugar-sweetened beverage tax on children, or the effect of the uses of the revenue generated. Since enacting the sugar-sweetened beverage tax, employment across the food sector in Berkeley increased by 7.2 percent and food-sector sales tax revenue increased approximately 15 percent (Silver, 2017). Taken together, the findings suggest that "taxes may be effective in shifting consumers to healthier beverages without undue economic hardship and while raising revenue," stated Silver.

Silver then described two models for warning labels proposed as local laws: labeling on products and labeling on print advertising. On-product labeling has yet to be passed as legislation, being defeated in California and in New York State. Warning labels on print advertisement, in contrast, would primarily affect point-of-sale ads in stores and on coolers. Warning labels on certain sugar-sweetened beverage print advertising has been passed in San Francisco, but it is currently being challenged in the courts. Two experimental studies suggest that adolescents and adults would be less likely to select sugar-sweetened beverages if the product carried a warning label (Roberto et al., 2016; VanEpps and Roberto, 2016). Silver also cited two international examples of warning labels. Chile uses a black octagon as a front-of-package warning on all foods with sugar over a certain level, and Ecuador uses a traffic light indicating the level of sugar, which has led to product reformulation.

"Building understanding, community support, and political feasibility is the greatest obstacle," said Silver. She believes that local strategies are likely to act synergistically—"it really is looking at how we pull different measures together." Silver concluded by saying she felt that the strategies to limit sugar-sweetened beverages are similar to how Tarja Halonen, former president of Finland, described smoke-free air—new ideas go from being ridiculous, to being possible, to being normal.

Legal Challenges to Limiting Sugar-Sweetened Beverages[6]

Mello began her remarks by noting that the local level is a source of innovative approaches to limit sugar-sweetened beverages, and that only a subset of these strategies have been legally challenged. While the plaintiffs vary and are typically individuals, she suggested that a variety of industry, restaurant, retail, and advertising groups and organizations are often behind the lawsuits. These lawsuits seek declaratory relief (a declaration that the law is illegal) and injunctive relief (an order to stop the law from taking effect).

Reflecting on lawsuits that have been brought against sugar-sweetened beverage ordinances, Mello noted that regulating commercial speech is

[6] This section summarizes information presented by Michelle Mello.

difficult from a legal perspective, technicalities in local and state laws are being leveraged by those challenging the laws, and legal challenges should be expected but can be overcome with careful planning.

Mello suggested that regulations on sugar-sweetened beverage advertisements are more difficult to legally defend than an outright ban on a product. She explained that what makes it so challenging is judicial protection of commercial speech. To highlight this point, Mello described a lawsuit brought against two San Francisco ordinances. One ordinance restricts the advertisement of sugar-sweetened beverages on certain city properties. The other is an ordinance that would require a warning label on sugar-sweetened beverage advertisements. Those in opposition to the two ordinances view them as restricting commercial speech while also forcing companies to express the government's viewpoint (compelled speech), said Mello. Decisions on such cases tend to come down to the stringency of the standard of judicial review—that is, how closely the court looks at the justification for the law, she stated. In cases of compelled speech, the government can get a quite favorable standard of review if it can demonstrate that it is merely requiring the disclosure of factual and uncontroversial information. In the case of the San Francisco warning label ordinance, the plaintiffs argue that the information is not uncontroversial because questions exist as to whether the health effects of added versus natural sugars are similar, and because there is disagreement about the specific contribution of sugar-sweetened beverages to the obesity epidemic, said Mello. She noted that it is not presently clear if the courts will require the disclosure to be uncontroversial, or merely accurate and factual. While there is precedent for courts to rule that disclosures need only be accurate and factual, but perhaps still scientifically controversial—as was the case for a recent case in Berkeley regarding cell phone radiation—Mello noted that it remains to be seen what standard of review will be applied in San Francisco.

On her second point, Mello provided three examples of how legal technicalities have been used to challenge various strategies to limit purchasing sugar-sweetened beverages. In the first example, she explained that the New York City portion cap was adopted by the Board of Health and was overturned because the City Charter only granted the City Council the authority to impose such a rule. In the case brought against the Philadelphia sugar-sweetened beverage tax, Mello noted that the objectors invoked a state law that restricts what taxes can be imposed at the local level (the Sterling Act), and argued that it was a duplicative tax. The third example she highlighted, also used in the challenge to the Philadelphia sugar-sweetened beverage tax, was the uniformity clause in the Pennsylvania Constitution, which requires taxes to be applied in a uniform way.

Mello concluded her remarks with the observation that many legal challenges to local public policy can be avoided through careful policy design decisions informed by legal guidance. She emphasized the importance of cities keeping a record of their decision making and documenting the science behind the policy so an adequate evidentiary basis underlies the legal defense.

PANEL DISCUSSION

Following Mello's presentation, Siega-Riz moderated a panel discussion that incorporated audience questions toward the end of the session. Siega-Riz opened the discussion by asking what partnerships have not yet been considered. Wootan responded by saying that partnerships are quite common in public health, and perhaps to a fault in certain circumstances. She thought that there are points in the process where not every stakeholder needs to be involved. Based on her experience with partnerships and advocacy, Wootan felt that different approaches can be used at different times to bring partners to the table. Mello noted that there are toolkits and guides to help communities navigate the legal defense of local strategies, and local attorneys could be an important resource for understanding the parameters of state laws. Silver noted that there could be two types of partnerships: public–private partnerships, as have been used for salt reduction, for example, and social partnerships (e.g., mobilized community partners), such as those used to pass sugar-sweetened beverage taxes over industry opposition. Which type of partnership is best to use, she noted, can depend on the context of the situation.

Siega-Riz next posed an audience member question that asked about the difference between warning labels for sugar-sweetened beverages and those on tobacco products. Mello replied that tobacco warning labels arose under the fairness doctrine, in which the Federal Communications Commission permits equal time to be allocated to opposing viewpoints on broadcast media. She stated that the tobacco industry did not fight this doctrine. Mello indicated that there is no analog to this doctrine for food. Wootan commented that policies initially perceived as controversial typically become acceptable, necessary, and inevitable over time through educating the public and raising awareness. Silver stated the evidence base of the risk and epidemiological relationship about sugar-sweetened beverages exists and can be part of a sound evidence base used as a legal defense for local ordinances; evidence on how much each intervention affects risk will take time to build.

Siega-Riz also asked the panelists to share what they thought could be learned from the Philadelphia sugar-sweetened beverage tax and what the next steps might be. Mello responded that the purpose of adopting the tax had nothing to do with preventing obesity or obesity-related illness, but instead was positioned to generate revenue. She explained that this positioning is why artificially sweetened beverages that have zero calories are included in Philadelphia's definition of sugar-sweetened beverages. Silver added that these measures will be much more successful if they are framed as generating revenue for something people care about. Wootan commented that the message that works is the message that best resonates with consumers. She rationalized that nobody wants increased taxes, but people do want health and child care.

In the final question posed to the panel, Siega-Riz asked the speakers to reflect on possible trickle-down effects of these regulations on children 5 years of age and younger. Silver explained that these policy efforts that are not specifically targeting young children will benefit children by changing the broader social and societal norms. Wootan thought that making low-fat milk or water the default beverage for young children at restaurants would help to create a habit that would follow children as they age.

6

The Role of Industry in Sugar-Sweetened Beverage Consumption

Moderator Barbara Devaney, senior fellow at Mathematica Policy Research, began by noting that the session would consider industry's role in current consumption patterns in the United States and explore approaches industry could take to reduce sugar-sweetened beverage consumption through approaches such as marketing, partnerships, product reformulation, and other strategies. Jennifer Harris, director of marketing initiatives at the Rudd Center for Food Policy and Obesity, spoke first, offering her perspective on marketing sugar-sweetened beverages to young children and their parents. Next, Richard Black, a principal at Quadrant D Consulting, outlined voluntary and regulatory industry approaches regarding sugar-sweetened beverages. Anne Ferree, the Alliance for a Healthier Generation's leader of engagement with the business sector, then described partnerships with industry to improve beverage choices for young children. A facilitated discussion with the audience, moderated by Devaney, followed the prepared remarks.

MARKETING SUGAR-SWEETENED BEVERAGES TO YOUNG CHILDREN AND THEIR PARENTS[1]

Harris provided definitions for key terms she used throughout her presentation in order to provide a common foundation:

[1] This section summarizes information presented by Jennifer Harris.

- *Sugar-sweetened beverages* was used to describe any beverage that contains added sugars (e.g., soda, fruit-flavored drinks),[2] including sweetened milks and supplements designed for very young children.
- *Marketing* was defined as "anything that influences people's purchases, attitudes, [and] opinions." Harris noted that marketing encompasses "product formulation, packaging, claims, promotions, licensed characters, shelf placement, point-of-sale displays," and other avenues.
- *Advertising* was defined as persuasive messages disseminated through mass media, such as television, radio, the Internet, and print.
- *Brand* was defined as the collection of images and concepts that represent the customer experience.

Citing a 2006 Institute of Medicine report on food marketing to children and youth (IOM, 2006), Harris explained that marketing affects children's "brand recall, preferences, requests to parents, and short-term consumption of advertised products." Since the release of the report, evidence has emerged to suggest that food advertising increases children's preference of a product category (e.g., advertising for a specific soda brand increases preference for soda in general), increases caloric consumption while viewing the advertisement, improves the perception of a product, normalizes a product, and makes the product appear appropriate and suited for children (Harris et al., 2009; Kelly et al., 2015).

Harris then discussed three broad topic areas: beverages marketed as intended for children, marketing and advertising beverages to children, and marketing beverages to parents.

Beverages Marketed as Intended for Children

Sugar-sweetened beverages that are marketed as intended for children are mostly fruit drinks and a few flavored waters (Harris et al., 2014). Harris showed that the nutrition profiles of such products remained relatively unchanged between 2011 and 2014 (see Table 6-1). She highlighted that approximately 40 percent of these products contain nonnutritive sweeteners, such as stevia or sucralose. Despite the proportion of products containing juice increasing between 2011 and 2014, the median juice content of such products remained the same—at 5 percent juice.

[2] In her presentation, Harris defined the term *sugary drinks*. As noted in Chapter 1, for consistency of language, the term *sugar-sweetened beverages* is used throughout this proceedings.

TABLE 6-1 Nutrition Profile of Children's Beverages, 2011 and 2014

	2011	2014
# of companies/brands	5/9	5/8
# of products	95	93
Calories per serving: median (range) calories	60 (10–120)	60 (10–130)
Sugar: median (range) grams	16 (2–29)	16 (2–33)
% of products with:		
Nonnutritive sweetener	40%	41%
Juice	32%	45%
Juice content (% of products with juice)	5% (5–11%)	5% (5–11%)

SOURCE: As presented by Jennifer Harris, June 22, 2017.

Marketing and Advertising Beverages to Children

Studies suggest that children younger than approximately 8 years of age view advertising as information and are not able to grasp its persuasive intent (IOM, 2006; Wilcox et al., 2004). It has therefore been argued that marketing to young children is inherently misleading (Harris and Graff, 2012; Pomeranz, 2010). Harris explained that companies use various approaches to market to young children, including attractive packaging, online games, and brand and licensed characters.

Shifting her remarks toward advertising, Harris discussed the voluntary Children's Food and Beverage Advertising Initiative (CFBAI). Implemented in 2007, CFBAI establishes nutrition standards for products whose advertising is directed primarily to children younger than 12 years of age. Most of the companies that participate in CFBAI also have a policy to refrain from directing advertising toward children younger than 6 years of age. Harris credited CFBAI for no full-sugar beverages being advertised on child-oriented television in 2016. She noted, however, that while advertising is not directly targeted at young children, children in this age range do encounter advertising when they watch programming that is viewed by a wide audience of children and adults. Furthermore, evidence suggests that black children are exposed to approximately 60 percent more food advertising than their white counterparts, partially due to watching more television.

Marketing Beverages to Parents

In explaining the marketing of children's beverages, Harris said:

> The strategy for children's products is really two-pronged. It's advertise to the kids to get them to ask their parents for the product, and then market to the parents to give them permission to purchase the product for their child.

One way in which children's beverages are marketed to parents is through nutrition claims (e.g., "good source of vitamin E"). Harris noted that, on average, children's beverages have 4.3 nutrition claims per package. Use of fruit images on packages and placement of a shelf-stable product next to orange juice in the refrigerated section in the grocery store are other examples Harris shared.

A survey of 1,100 parents provided insight into the opinions and behaviors of parents regarding various beverages. Results found that 92 percent with a child 2 to 5 years of age provided some form of sugar-sweetened beverage in the month prior to the survey (Munsell et al., 2016). On average, 2.4 different types of beverages were provided, with 80 percent serving fruit drinks, approximately one-third providing flavored waters and sports drinks, and 40 percent providing soda. Parents who provided sugar-sweetened beverages were more likely to view such products as very or somewhat healthy, as compared to parents who did not provide such beverages. Parents also tended to view particular brands as healthier than the product category.

Harris also shared unpublished data on child beverage sales, particularly single-serving bottles and aseptic juices. Of the child-targeted beverages, 71 percent contained added sugars, as compared to 46 percent of other products. Sales of child-targeted products with added sugars were also more responsive to price reductions than other products and child-targeted products with no sweeteners. Promotional displays had a similar effect, noted Harris.

To conclude her presentation, Harris drew attention to toddler drinks (also called toddler milks or toddler formulas), a fairly new product category with the intended consumer being young children who no longer consume infant formula. The marketing of such products largely focuses on benefits to children's growth and development. Harris noted that all toddler drinks currently on the market have structure/function claims (a claim suggesting an ingredient will be beneficial to the child in some way), averaging 2.3 claims per package. Total advertising spending on toddler drinks has increased since 2011, whereas it has decreased for infant formulas (see Figure 6-1). Harris noted that toddler drinks are heavily advertised in Spanish-language media. Referring to these products as "sweetened milk," Harris characterized toddler drinks as an emerging issue.

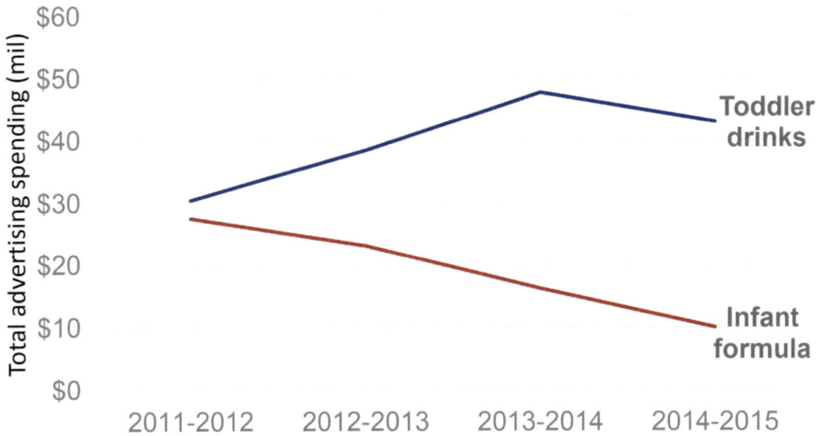

FIGURE 6-1 Advertising spending on infant formula and toddler drinks.
SOURCE: As presented by Jennifer Harris, June 22, 2017.

SUGAR-SWEETENED BEVERAGES: VOLUNTARY AND REGULATORY INDUSTRY APPROACHES[3]

Black's presentation focused on four central topics: establishing trust, interpreting statistics, building on successes and acknowledging failures, and considering impediments and opportunities for forward progress.

Establishing Trust

"Simply because you work in one space or another does not mean you should not be trusted," stated Black. Trust among stakeholders is essential to forward progress. Drawing on the definitions of Solomon and Flores (2001), Black presented trust as a spectrum. Blind trust, an unwavering type of trust that continues even in spite of betrayal, anchors one end of the spectrum. Simple trust follows and is a type of trust that lacks doubt, but may not be restored if betrayed. At the other end of the spectrum is a "façade of goodwill and congeniality that hides distrust" called cordial hypocrisy, a type of trust that impedes honest communication. Authentic trust exists in the middle of the spectrum. Underlying authentic trust is an awareness that disappointment and betrayal are possibilities, and as such, authentic trust is something that must be fostered. Black explained that the food and

[3] This section summarizes information presented by Richard Black.

BOX 6-1
Seven Features of Successful Partnerships

- A sense of authentic trust
- Mutuality (working toward a common goal, with the benefits of achieving that goal being different for different partners)
- The feasibility of achieving the desired outcome
- Joint planning
- The formulation of clear procedural steps for risk mitigation
- The establishment of general project management processes
- Complementarity (all partners contributing unique, but complementary resources)

SOURCE: As presented by Richard Black, June 22, 2017.

beverage industries seek to establish and cultivate authentic trust through partnerships and highlighted features that make for successful partnerships (see Box 6-1). He emphasized that while biases need to be acknowledged and managed, "everyone brings something worthwhile to the table."

Interpreting Statistics

Black demonstrated the need for careful interpretation of statistics by first using an example of advertising to children. He stated that television advertisement is considered child-directed if 30 percent or more of the program's audience are children, irrespective of total viewership. A television show with a large audience could remain under the 30 percent threshold while drawing a greater absolute number of children as compared to children's programming with a smaller total audience. Black pointed out that while children see advertisements, as it is currently determined, they are not targeted in general.

To further emphasize his point, Black presented a graph showing the prevalence of adult obesity increasing between 1999 and 2009, while the daily per capita calories from sugar-sweetened beverages were decreasing during the same period. Layering on the context of consumption patterns (see Figure 6-2), he indicated that the per capita data encompass a situation in which the top quartile of the population is consuming the majority of a product and overconsumption persists. He drew a parallel with per capita sugar-sweetened beverage intake in India and Latin America, in which intake in India is less and could be interpreted as a nonissue. The data from India, a country in which most of the population lives in rural

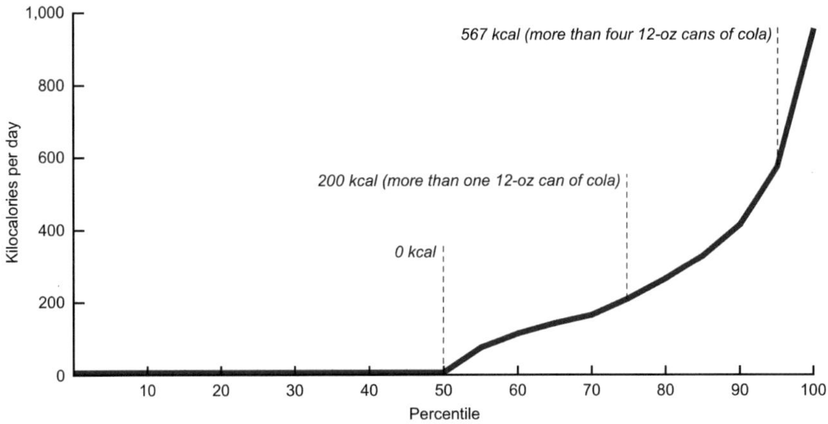

FIGURE 6-2 Sugar-sweetened beverage consumption on a given day for Americans 2 years of age and older based on 2005–2008 National Health and Nutrition Examination Survey data.
SOURCES: As presented by Richard Black, June 22, 2017; Ogden et al., 2011.

settings, reveal that the majority of intake is occurring in urban areas, noted Black. In thinking about impact, he suggested that the focus needs to be on understanding who is consuming sugar-sweetened beverages.

Building on Successes and Acknowledging Failures

Next, Black discussed voluntary efforts in which industry has engaged to address sugar-sweetened beverage consumption. A partnership with the Clinton Foundation, for example, led to the beverage industry agreeing to voluntarily eliminate full-calorie beverages from schools and follow guidelines for elementary, middle, and high schools. Subsequent to this agreement, calories shipped to U.S. schools decreased by 90 percent. Through the Healthy Weight Commitment Foundation, industry members have removed more than 6 trillion calories per year from the marketplace, exceeding its initial goal of 1.5 trillion calories.

Black used predictive models of the Healthy Weight Commitment Foundation calorie goal to again highlight challenges of interpreting data. One of the predictive models (a negatively accelerating curve) suggested the calorie reduction in the marketplace followed as expected, where another predictive model (linear time trend) suggested the reductions that took place were much greater than expected. Black's point was not to argue the merits of the models, but instead to emphasize the importance of considering different perspectives.

Other voluntary initiatives taken by industry have included placing calorie information on the front of packages and reformulating and developing products to be lower in calories. Black noted that there have been attempts to reformulate existing sugar-sweetened beverages to have lower calorie content, but it continues to be a challenge owing, in part, to consumer expectation and acceptability. He acknowledged that not all consumers are receptive to health messages and, as such, there is not a "one size fits all" solution.

Black drew attention to what he perceives is a limitation of existing excise taxes on sugar-sweetened beverages. Using the tax in Mexico as an example, he highlighted that the existing taxes are graduated based on the volume of the product, which does not provide an incentive to companies to lower sugar content of the taxed products. He suggested that a graduated tax based on grams of sugar would incentivize such reductions. Black cited that analyses from Mexico indicate that per capita sugar-sweetened beverage consumption had significantly decreased after instituting the tax, but that consumption of taxed carbonated sodas has decreased less than their noncarbonated taxed counterparts.

Considering Impediments to and Opportunities for Forward Progress

With more than 3 billion people having access to the Internet and approximately 60 percent of the global population having access to a personal mobile device, Black expressed that there is an opportunity to better leverage digital media. He also emphasized the need to have countervailing voices to refute misinformation. Black concluded by saying that accountability is a key aspect of partnerships—for creating and meeting targets that can be measured and interpreted—and that partners need to be active supporters of such efforts.

PARTNERSHIPS WITH INDUSTRY TO IMPROVE BEVERAGE CHOICES OF YOUNG CHILDREN[4]

The Alliance for a Healthier Generation (hereafter referred to as the Alliance) was established in 2005 as a joint initiative of the American Heart Association and the Clinton Foundation. The Alliance strives to create healthier community environments and to work with companies to transform the marketplace in an effort to improve children's health. To create a systemic change, the work of the Alliance extends beyond just the marketplace, and includes efforts in schools, after-school programs, summer camps, early care and education settings, and juvenile justice facilities.

[4] This section summarizes information presented by Anne Ferree.

Because there is no single cause for the health issues children face, noted Ferree, there cannot be a single solution.

Ferree provided an overview of the 2006 Alliance School Beverage Guidelines, which was the first agreement between the Alliance and the business sector. The voluntary guidelines, which predated the Healthy, Hunger-Free Kids Act of 2010, were brokered with the American Beverage Association, the Coca-Cola Company, PepsiCO, and Cadbury-Schweppes (now Dr. Pepper-Snapple). Ferree explained that through the partnership, companies agreed to a number of changes, including phasing out sales of full-calorie carbonated soft drinks, shifting product combinations to favor low- and no-calorie beverages, and reducing portion sizes of products sold in schools. The Alliance had an independent, third-party evaluator assess the effect of the agreement. Between 2004 and the 2009–2010 school year, beverage calories shipped to schools decreased by 90 percent; volume of beverages shipped to schools decreased by 77 percent; volume of full-calorie, carbonated soft drinks shipped to schools decreased by 97 percent; and volume of restricted beverages (including juice drinks, flavored water, and teas) shipped to schools decreased by 94 percent (Wescott et al., 2012).

Ferree explained that the Alliance believes that there is "a place at the table for every single company in this country," large or small, and she shared lessons her organization has learned through its range of partnerships across various sectors. First, Ferree emphasized the importance of taking a systems approach to researching an issue, identifying gaps, and considering solutions. As an example, she showed a diagram of the various elements of the food system (e.g., food production, distribution and aggregation, marketing, preparation and consumption), and stated that trying to understand the issues to the fullest extent possible helps in the identification of companies to engage.

Ferree then noted that there is no single approach to developing meaningful and impactful partnerships. The Alliance has found success by engaging entire sectors, and she noted that finding a shared value is a foundational step to forming such relationships. She acknowledged that collaboration with companies in the same sector can be complex, and it requires attention to issues of confidentiality, accountability, and impartiality. When an entire sector is not amenable to coming to the table at one time, the Alliance intentionally structures agreements with companies with the largest market share to create a domino effect. Such an approach was taken in the Alliance's efforts to improve children's menus. Ferree said, "Sometimes one large company can make such a difference that [it is] worth going ahead and working with them in a really concerted way." Another key to the Alliance's enduring partnerships has been seeking top-down backing from "high-level champions" within the partner companies, Ferree stated. To that end, she emphasized the importance of understanding where a business is coming from and to being able to "speak their language." Because public health issues are not constantly at the forefront of their partners' minds, and shareholder monetary value is, Ferree explained that the Alliance brings that knowledge and challenges the thinking of their partners.

Ferree emphasized the value of maintaining transparency and preserving integrity over the lifetime of a partnership. The Alliance has included having a credible, third-party, nongovernmental organization involved from the beginning to set goals and determine how the agreement will be evaluated and communicated, as well as retaining an evaluator to not only verify that each agreement is being executed, but also to measure the results of each agreement.

Changing consumer behavior toward products with less sugar and fewer calories has been challenging, Ferree remarked. She said that the Alliance's second agreement with the beverage industry, which is built on long-term relationships, has a goal of reducing beverage calories consumed per person per day in the United States by 20 percent by 2025 (from 199 calories per day in 2014, to 159 calories per day by 2025). Through the agreement, partners will:

- Continue to promote calorie and sugar awareness on all company-owned equipment, which includes millions of vending machines, retail coolers, and fountains in convenience stores, restaurants, and other locations.
- Transform consumer palates through innovating, reformulating, distributing, and marketing no- and low-calorie beverages.
- Create incentives and engagement through consumer education and outreach at the community level.

Ferree added that the companies are also engaging in work in 8 to 10 communities to test and learn what works in creating the desired shifts. Ferree concluded her presentation by reminding the audience that engaging the business sector is about individual relationship building, trust building, understanding their business, and finding a common goal.

FACILITATED DISCUSSION WITH THE AUDIENCE

Following Ferree's presentation, she, Black, and Harris took part in a facilitated discussion with the audience, moderated by Devaney. Topics that emerged during the conversation included unintended consequences, marketing and advertising, use of technology, and partnerships.

Unintended Consequences

Devaney opened the discussion by asking the speakers to broadly discuss the possibility of unintended consequences as a result of any of the strategies. Harris explained that the focus of CFBAI was on advertising to children younger than 12 years of age and that after it was implemented, advertising to children 12 to 17 years of age dramatically increased. As another example, Harris thought that there may be unintended consequences of some of the healthy children's meal initiatives. She suggested that fewer parents are buying children's meals for their children. "I'm afraid we may be pushing parents to the cheaper, but less nutritious higher-calorie options on the menu," stated Harris. She also noted that as sugar is going down in the beverages, the artificial sweeteners or the nonnutritive sweeteners are being added. Harris felt that the topic of artificial sweeteners is an area where the nutrition community needs to weigh in, and perhaps more disclosure about what is in the products is needed.

In response to Devaney's question, Ferree reminded the audience that one of the challenges is that beverage companies and restaurants react to the wants of the customer. She explained that the Alliance's most recent beverage agreement included 100 percent juice as part of the goal because an unintended consequence of earlier initiatives to reduce soda consumption may have led to increases in consumption of 100 percent juice. Black thought that an unintended consequence of Philadelphia's tax is that it does not incentivize the companies to change, as it is applied to all sweetened beverages. He suggested that the tax might potentially fail to maximize the opportunity for behavioral change.

Later in the session, Devaney posed an audience member question, specifically asking about unintended consequences related to product reformulation. Harris replied, there are brand managers who are responsible for profit across all products within their brands and their goal is to increase sales for all of those products. She stated that a recommendation made in a Healthy Eating Research report was that if a product is marketed on children's television, all the products within that brand should meet the nutrition standards that are set. Ferree pointed out that another way of thinking about it is to incentivize companies to incrementally introduce products that are lower in calories and eventually replace the higher-calorie, higher-sugar products.

Suggesting that it could possibly be an unintended consequence, Devaney asked the speakers if juice concentrates are being used in place of other sweeteners. Black expressed his concerns over "stripped" juice concentrates, which, in his view, are indistinguishable from sugar water because the characterizing aspects of the juice, and likely the beneficial components, have been removed. Ferree responded that the Alliance focuses on all calories and all sugars, in an effort to avoid the swapping of one caloric sweetener for another. An audience member, identified as a representative from the Juice Products Association, said that if a juice concentrate is reconstituted to the Brix level of 100 percent juice, it is not considered a sweetener, but if the juice concentrate is added to a product to sweeten and not reconstituted to its 100 percent level, then it would be considered a sweetener.

Marketing and Advertising

Devaney combined several audience member questions to ask the speakers about differences in the effects of marketing by race, ethnicity, or socioeconomic status, and the consistency of efforts to reduce advertising across population groups. Harris replied that there has been limited research to date regarding the effects of marketing on different population groups. She described one hypothesis that currently exists: advertising portrays images of the world that are aspirational for lower-income individuals or recent immigrants, and, as such, would be more effective with those audiences. Harris also noted that targeted marketing to black or Hispanic audiences—groups who have not been traditionally reflected in advertising—appears to be creating goodwill and could potentially be more effective. Disparities in exposure to advertising between black and white youths are growing, Harris noted. Exposure appears to be decreasing for white youths but remaining unchanged for black youths, she elaborated.

An audience member asked the speakers if the definition of child-targeted marketing should be changed. Harris explained that there is a fair amount of marketing not covered by CFBAI. She added that a HER report recommended that CFBAI's definition of children be extended to include children up to 14 years of age and be applied to television programming viewed by this age group. Harris added that First Amendment issues arise when such restrictions are applied to television programs with a sizable adult audience.

One audience member proposed replacing advertising for sugar-sweetened beverages with advertising for more nutrient-dense beverages and healthier food choices. Harris responded that the 2006 Institute of Medicine food marketing to children report recommended that companies use their creativity and resources to market healthier foods to children in place of the unhealthy food that is typically advertised (IOM, 2006). This recommendation has long been discussed, but has yet to be executed, she noted. Harris acknowledged that foods, such as fruits, vegetables, and milk do not have the profit margins that packaged processed foods do. She also said there is also the philosophical question—should children be advertised to at all? She acknowledged that parents ultimately decide what to serve their children, and reiterated that young children's cognitive abilities really are not developed enough to understand the marketing. Drawing on an idea he credited to Hank Cardello, Black suggested that the tax deduction for advertising expenses could be reduced for less healthy foods so it is more expensive for the company to advertise, and conversely the tax deduction could be increased for the healthier food items.

Use of Technology

When asked if there are specific success stories of how technology or social media is used to improve food and beverage consumption, Black responded that one person, owing to the platform of the Internet, can actually cause a company to respond and change. He said that campaigns have sped up the rate or the pace at which companies respond, but can also be a platform for exaggeration and misinformation. Harris indicated that the food industry has been at the forefront of digital and social media marketing. She acknowledged that viral social media campaigns are a low-cost approach that can have an effect. Black added, "The beauty of the Internet is that you [do not] need money, you need creativity."

An audience member asked the speakers if it was possible to have an intervention that would give parents the ability to control their children's exposure to advertisements. Harris suggested that parents monitor and track what websites their children are visiting. She added that children should only be exposed to high-quality media, such as noncommercial media.

Partnerships

Devaney posed a question from the audience regarding federal involvement in partnerships. Ferree said that she did not know about federal support specifically, but indicated that there is a role for government (e.g., local departments of health) so there is alignment of messages and campaigns. Black stated that the examples tend to be more on the research side, as opposed to outreach and consumer education. He noted that the International Life Sciences Institute, for example, led an initiative with the U.S. Department of Agriculture (USDA) to develop a branded foods database. At present, the database is populated with approximately 200,000 branded foods and is used for the dietary assessment portion of the National Health and Nutrition Examination Survey. He explained that the food industry supplies the data. From the audience, Robert Post added that the MyPlate strategic partners' effort with the USDA Center for Nutrition Policy and Program serves as an example. Through this partnership, he elaborated, MyPlate programming is used by more than 100 large multisector organizations.

In thinking about partnership, an audience member asked the speakers if changes in consumption of sugar-sweetened beverages should be considered the measure of success. Ferree responded that, ideally, measurements would be taken in different ways (e.g., changes in consumption, across product type, in availability) to really understand what is having an effect, but she acknowledged that it is not always feasible, primarily because it is resource intensive. Black said he is in favor of using very specific measures and suggested that the measure to limit sugar-sweetened beverages is straightforward.

7

Reflections and an Exploration of Gaps and Opportunities

The last session of the workshop reflected on and summarized key messages from the preceding sessions, explored the evidence and research needs that exist, and considered opportunities to fill the identified gaps. To achieve these objectives, Virginia Stallings, professor of pediatrics at the University of Pennsylvania Perelman School of Medicine and director of the Nutrition Center at the Children's Hospital of Philadelphia, was charged with providing her reflections on the material that had been presented over the course of the day and a half workshop. She then moderated a panel discussion, which expanded to a facilitated discussion toward the end of the session. Panelists included Richard Black, Stephen Daniels, Marlene Schwartz, and Mary Story. At the end of the discussion, Karen Weber Cullen provided brief, concluding remarks.

REFLECTIONS ON THE WORKSHOP[1]

To begin her reflections, Stallings reminded the audience of the workshop's age group of interest—children from birth to 5 years of age. She thought the broad information that had been presented during the workshop, which encompassed older children and adults, showcased that "there is so little information and so little specificity" for infants, toddlers, and preschool-age children. Young children are not customers and are completely dependent on what is served or offered to them. Stallings perceived this as a strength of focusing on children 5 years of age and younger, and is

[1] This section summarizes information presented by Virginia Stallings.

something that could be leveraged. Young children are provided beverages in settings beyond just the home environment. As such, Stallings emphasized the importance of engaging not only parents, but also other caretakers across the spectrum of child care settings.

In discussing the role of federal nutrition programs, Stallings pointed to changes to the food packages offered through the Special Supplemental Nutrition Program for Women, Infants, and Children (WIC), as well as school meals and competitive food policies, as examples of improvements that have been made. From her perspective, similar opportunities for change currently exist for the Supplemental Nutrition Assistance Program and, to a lesser extent, the Child and Adult Care Feeding Program (CACFP). Stallings also raised the issue of a lack of federal policy for children ranging from birth to 24 months of age. She noted that this gap has been primarily filled by public statements on infant and child feeding practices from the American Academy of Pediatrics. The gap has the potential to be filled through the work of the B-24 Project, and it is within the authority of the *2020–2025 Dietary Guidelines for Americans* to provide guidance for this age group.

Identifying portion size as a key issue, Stallings said, "There is an inherent difficulty in portion sizes with liquids that we have to think about. You can drink a lot of calories very fast." One of the challenges related to portion size mentioned by Stallings is that cups, even sippy cups, are often larger than 4 ounces. Another consideration she raised was the role of economic value and incentives to consume more (e.g., free refills), particularly for those in poverty.

Stallings then reflected on specific types of beverages. She suggested that while whole fruit is preferential, 100 percent juice still has a place in the dietary pattern when provided within age-appropriate portion sizes. Stallings expressed that the approach to handling 100 percent juice in the diet merits its own separate discussions. There are also issues related to drinking water, both broadly and as they specifically relate to this age group. For example, there is currently ambiguity regarding whether or not water should be given to children younger than 12 months of age. Other issues Stallings highlighted included "having safe water, creating a culture in the United States where water is the next beverage that you might give young children," and differentiating between plain and flavored non-caloric water. In considering beverage consumption of young children from a broad perspective, Stallings offered, "There are some things that we, as a culture, recognize are appropriate for children of this age. For example, we believe a few things are adult beverages. Alcohol, coffee—generally those are not things you are going to want someone under 5 to have."

To conclude, Stallings remarked that there are opportunities to recast the goal of limiting consumption of sugar-sweetened beverages by young children into a "public health step and message that all parents and communities and even the government can be proud of." She noted there are several examples of initiatives that have communicated public health messages to families, and pointed to examples such as choking hazards in first foods and sleeping positions for the prevention of sudden infant death syndrome. To achieve a similar effect with sugar-sweetened beverages, Stallings urged the audience to think through ways to define the message, work on building a strong evidence base, enhance cultural awareness, and become relevant to individuals across all socioeconomic groups. She also pointed out the range of roles that government, from local to federal, could play by using tools such as executive orders and City Council decisions that include revising regulations around the availability of sugar-sweetened beverages to participants in nutrition assistance programs and the importance of looking to the food industry to develop new products. "Stakeholders, partners, community—all of those—are really essential to getting this done," she said. Stallings said that it is a goal to bring the birth to 24-month age group into the public health domain and reduce sugar-sweetened beverage consumption as a part of public health programs.

PANEL DISCUSSION

After her prepared remarks, Stallings moderated a panel discussion with Black, Daniels, Schwartz, and Story. The discussed topics were initially drawn from brief statements made by each of the panelists and from questions provided by the audience in the facilitated discussion format. Toward the end of the session, questions were taken directly from the audience members in an active question-and-answer format. The sections below summarize the topics that emerged over the course of the panel discussion.

Brief Statements from Each of the Panelists

To begin, each panelist gave a brief statement about what they perceived were key topic areas for discussion. In reflecting on the Session 1 presentations and in citing a recent dietary intake analysis among children 2 to 19 years of age in the United States (Rosinger et al., 2017), Story indicated that sugar-sweetened beverage consumption is pervasive among youths and a need exists to intervene while children are young. To target children from birth to 5 years of age, Story suggested that the focus needs to be on juice-flavored drinks (also known as juice drinks, juice beverages, nectars, fruit drinks) that are not 100 percent fruit juice.

During his remarks, Black emphasized two concepts. First, he discussed sugar-sweetened beverage taxes, cautioning against trying to regulate sweetness, and suggesting that it would be ideal to target the amount of added sugars. Second, he highlighted the importance of identifying partners, including those who are "not the usual suspects."

A dietary pattern approach is needed to help guide how to optimize intake, Daniels reflected, because young children are currently consuming an excess of calories while not consuming sufficient amounts of many nutrients. He also offered that one strategy to consider is finding better ways to implement guidelines.

Schwartz discussed research needs related to 100 percent juice and flavored milk. She suggested that there is "an empirical question about what would happen if we really recommended that [children] not drink 100 percent fruit juice up until age 5," and she recognized that there is uncertainty about the possible forms of juice substitutes that parents or caregivers might choose. Her group recently conducted a 2-year study on the effects of removing flavored milk from schools and found consumption of plain milk increased over time (Schwartz et al., 2017). Additional research is needed, she noted, especially on the longitudinal effect of removing flavored milk from preschools, kindergartens, and elementary schools on plain milk intake.

Fruit Drinks and 100 Percent Fruit Juice

Among the challenges discussed by the panel was the terminology used to characterize fruit drinks that are less than 100 percent juice. Schwartz suggested that describing such products as fruit drinks can lead to confusion since the term *fruit* is used, a sentiment shared by Story. Daniels questioned whether the term *fruit* might be reserved exclusively to describe 100 percent juice. One concern that could result from that kind of proposal, Black suggested, is that some specific terminologies that are used for flavor descriptions (e.g., *fruity*) do not meet the requirement for content claims as set forth by U.S. regulatory agencies. Instead of attempting to change the terminology, he proposed mandating that any fruit image be proportionate to the fruit content of the product, an approach that is currently being used in Canada.

A member of the audience noted that for a product to be considered "juice," it is required by law to be 100 percent juice, whereas a juice drink requires minimal juice content, but is required to put the percent juice on the container. Schwartz noted that this is what was so challenging about trying to teach parents the difference—it requires reading the ingredient list to understand the difference. She showed an example of how this information is labeled on a selection of products. Recognizing the complexities inherent in describing fruit drinks, Story advanced the notion of organizing a meeting or taskforce to consider how best to specify the description of these products and then leverage that as a means toward limiting their consumption by young children.

Dietary Intake of Infants and Longitudinal Data

The panel discussed the role and need for data, particularly in infants. Black wondered if it was necessary to collect data on children from birth to 6 months of age, as it is presumed that infants do not consume sugar-sweetened beverages. Stallings contested this idea, noting that "sometimes the prioritization or the imperative nature of change comes out of finding out something we [did not] believe was happening is happening." Daniels also challenged Black's comment, stating that longitudinal data are necessary in order to better understand how taste preferences develop in context of parental feeding habits and behaviors. With respect to longitudinal data, an audience member noted that the Food and Nutrition Service is currently conducting the WIC Infant and Toddler Feeding Practices Study II, and published its first report at the beginning of January (May et al., 2017).

A member of the audience asked if there were longitudinal data on the long-term effects of restricting young children's access to sugar-sweetened beverages; for instance, would young children drink more if they had the liberty to make their own drink selections? Leann Birch, moderator of the first session of the workshop, commented from the audience that there are analyses of data from the follow-up to the Infant Feeding Practices Study II (IFPS II) indicating that intake of sugar-sweetened beverages during infancy increased the likelihood of sugar-sweetened beverage consumption at 6 years of age. On the topic of restrictions, Black wondered if anything could be learned by the messages of industries that currently have such restrictions (e.g., alcohol). Stallings repeated the sentiment she expressed in her reflections—that there are beverages that are culturally accepted as inappropriate for young children—and thought this may be an area in which partnerships could potentially be explored.

Developing Effective Messages and Promoting Change Within Specific Population Groups

The panel also discussed ideas about developing effective messages. Messages about growth, health, and development, such as those being used to market toddler drinks, are significant to parents of young children, noted Schwartz. She later commented that the messaging about when to introduce water into an infant's diet needs to be clarified and done in such a way that is "very deliberate and intentional." Story noted that tailoring the message is crucial to fostering change within a particular population group. As an example, she pointed to a Session 4 presentation, in which

Henrietta Sandoval-Soland described using the phrase "water is sacred" in the Navajo Nation.

Black thought celebrities and cutting-edge approaches with social media could be leveraged. In such engagement, he suggested it is important to communicate a message that allows people to identify what products they want, rather than focusing on the products they are not supposed to have. In response to Black's comments, Stallings drew a parallel to the Got Milk? campaign. Later in the discussions, Black offered that "I [do not] think it's a big leap to get [celebrities] who are passionate about nutrition, broadly speaking, to say you can have a really big impact if you focus over here and work with us on this other aspect." A member of the audience commented that there could be learning and evidence from the U.S. Food and Drug Administration's tobacco control Real Cost campaign. The audience member noted that some of the focus group feedback on the subsequent Fresh Empire campaign emphasized the importance of the authenticity of the messenger. Another example the audience member suggested considering is the Truth campaign, which was funded by the tobacco Master Settlement Agreement and leveraged social media. Drawing on the audience member's point, Christina Hecht emphasized the importance of the funding required for advertisement and questioned who would be the champion for water. She noted that this presents an opportunity for creativity.

The discussion also explored the concept of food as a reward. Black suggested that sugar-sweetened beverages may serve as an accessible treat that low-income families can afford, and that strategies to reduce sugar-sweetened beverages need to provide opportunities for treats with less added sugars. Expanding on this idea, Stallings offered that one of the challenges is that food and beverages are part of our ceremonies, celebrations, and culture. Daniels added that he thought "we may not be challenging the concept of food as a reward enough." He continued by suggesting that a better understanding of food as a reward paradigm "would allow us to think about better strategies to deal with it." One idea would be to determine how to redirect rewards toward something that promotes child development, such as reading, Stallings proposed.

Leveraging the Child and Adult Feeding Program

An audience member asked the panelists whether states or cities should be providing more support to the programs that participate in CACFP to improve limitations of sugar-sweetened beverages. Story said that providing more support for such programs was a good idea. Black expressed that it is essential for such programs to agree on the measurable outcomes from the beginning and track efficacy. In revisiting this concept later in the discussion, an audience member made several points regarding CACFP and the potential for partnerships. She noted that CACFP is a suitable partner because it serves half of all early care and education settings and that approximately three-quarters of children served are from low-income families. CACFP has a best practice rule, taking effect in October 2017, which will reduce sugar-sweetened beverages. The audience member also suggested that partnerships between state and localities and CACFP could be beneficial when it comes to changing policies.

Milk Alternatives

An audience member asked the panel about educating the public about milk alternatives (e.g., soy milk, almond milk, coconut milk). Daniels questioned the use of milk alternatives among children 1 to 5 years of age, and expressed that he thought moving children away from cow's milk consumption was a mistake. While cow's milk protein allergies exist, he noted, they are relatively uncommon. Black wondered if this product category, at about 6 grams of sugar per serving, had a high enough sugar content to make it worthwhile to limit. Later in the session, Esa Davis, moderator of the second session of the workshop, suggested that there might be misperceptions about the prevalence of lactose intolerance and milk allergies that are absorbed by the community at large.

Engaging Health Care Providers

The panel also discussed strategies to help pediatricians, family practice physicians, oral health providers, and other health care providers reinforce the message regarding sugar-sweetened beverages. Daniels described nutrition education for medical students and residents as "woefully inadequate." Later, Ferree described the efforts on this front by the Alliance for a Healthier Generation, which include working alongside the the American Academy of Pediatrics, the Bipartisan Policy Center, and a number of other partners to transform the training systems used not only in medical schools, but also in all affiliated health care professional training systems. From the audience, Leann Birch emphasized the role of and opportunities to use WIC as a conduit for reaching parents.

CLOSING REMARKS

In her closing remarks, Cullen revisited the concept she presented to open the workshop. She noted that over the course of a day, a child may be in the care of a variety of caretakers in various surroundings, and that various influences affect what beverages are offered to and consumed by the child. She thought the strategies highlighted over the course of this workshop addressed the breadth of approaches currently available to limit sugar-sweetened beverage consumption. Reiterating points made during the preceding panel discussion, Cullen emphasized the importance of identifying a champion or someone with authentic representation of the different groups in order to effectively deliver and tailor the message. She also touched on the role of nutrition education through federal programs. Evidence gaps currently exist, Cullen noted, and include longitudinal studies of dietary patterns of children from birth to 5 years of age and studies exploring the effect of marketing on young children's consumption of sugar-sweetened beverages. She emphasized the role of family, but explained that misperceptions, behaviors, and beliefs may be barriers to limiting sugar-sweetened beverages in homes. Cullen suggested that a need exists to reduce these barriers and social norms around sugar-sweetened beverages.

References

AAP (American Academy of Pediatrics). 2011. *Nutrition: What every parent needs to know, second edition*. Elk Grove Village, IL: American Academy of Pediatrics.

AAP, American Public Health Association, and National Resource Center for Health and Safety in Child Care and Early Education. 2011. *Caring for our children: National health and safety performance standards; guidelines for early care and education programs. 3rd edition*. Elk Grove Village, IL: American Academy of Pediatrics.

AAP Committee on Nutrition. 2013. *Pediatric nutrition, 7th edition*. Elk Grove Village, IL: American Academy of Pediatrics.

Andreyeva, T., J. Luedicke, A. S. Tripp, and K. E. Henderson. 2013. Effects of reduced juice allowances in food packages for the Women, Infants, and Children Program. *Pediatrics* 131(5):919–927.

Anzman-Frasca, S., M. P. Mueller, S. Sliwa, P. R. Dolan, L. Harelick, S. B. Roberts, K. Washburn, and C. D. Economos. 2015. Changes in children's meal orders following healthy menu modifications at a regional U.S. restaurant chain. *Obesity (Silver Spring)* 23(5):1055–1062.

Arsenault, B. J., B. Lamarche, and J. P. Despres. 2017. Targeting overconsumption of sugar-sweetened beverages vs. overall poor diet quality for cardiometabolic diseases risk prevention: Place your bets! *Nutrients* 9(6):E600.

Baby-Friendly USA, Inc. 2012. Baby-Friendly USA. https://www.babyfriendlyusa.org (accessed September 27, 2017).

Baca, K. 2017. *NB3 beverage summit: "Decolonize" soda consumption, promote drinking water*. https://indiancountrymedianetwork.com/culture/health-wellness/we-have-to-make-water-cool-again-nb3-summit-fights-sugary-drinks (accessed August 23, 2017).

Bender, M. S., P. R. Nader, C. Kennedy, and S. Gahagan. 2013. A culturally appropriate intervention to improve health behaviors in Hispanic mother-child dyads. *Childhood Obesity* 9(2):157–163.

Britten, P., L. E. Cleveland, K. L. Koegel, K. J. Kuczynski, and S. M. Nickols-Richardson. 2012. Impact of typical rather than nutrient-dense food choices in the U.S. Department of Agriculture food patterns. *Journal of the Academy of Nutrition and Dietetics* 112(10):1560–1569.

Burgermaster, M., H. Bhana, M. D. Fullwood, D. A. Luna Bazaldua, and E. Tipton. 2017. Exploring the role of sugar-sweetened beverage consumption in obesity among New Yorkers using propensity score matching. *Journal of the Academy of Nutrition and Dietetics* 117(5):753–762.

CDC (Centers for Disease Control and Prevention). 2011. School health guidelines to promote healthy eating and physical activity. *Morbidity and Mortality Weekly Report Recommendations and Reports* 60(RR-5):1–76.

CDC. 2013. *Community health media center.* https://nccd.cdc.gov/chmc/Apps/overview.aspx (accessed August 21, 2017).

CDC. 2014a. *Increasing access to drinking water and other healthier beverages in early care and education settings.* Atlanta, GA: U.S. Department of Health and Human Services.

CDC. 2014b. *Increasing access to drinking water in schools.* Atlanta, GA: U.S. Department of Health and Human Services.

CDC. 2016a. *Comprehensive framework for addressing the school nutrition environment and services.* Atlanta, GA: U.S. Department of Health and Human Services.

CDC. 2016b. *Early care and education state indicator report, 2016.* https://www.cdc.gov/obesity/strategies/ece-state-indicator-report.html (accessed September 27, 2017).

CDC. n.d. *Spectrum of opportunities for obesity prevention in the early care and education setting.* https://www.cdc.gov/obesity/downloads/spectrum-of-opportunities-for-obesity-prevention-in-early-care-and-education-setting_tabriefing.pdf (accessed August 1, 2017).

Child Care Aware of America. 2017. *Child care in America: 2016 state fact sheets.* http://usa.childcareaware.org/wp-content/uploads/2016/07/2016-Fact-Sheets-Full-Report-02-27-17.pdf (accessed August 22, 2017).

Chriqui, J. F., F. J. Chaloupka, L. M. Powell, and S. S. Eidson. 2013. A typology of beverage taxation: Multiple approaches for obesity prevention and obesity prevention-related revenue generation. *Journal of Public Health Policy* 34(3):403–423.

Contra Costa Child Care Council. 2017. *C.H.O.I.C.E. toolkit and self-assessment questionnaire.* https://www.cocokids.org/child-health-nutrition/c-h-o-i-c-e-toolkit-self-assessment-questionnnaire (accessed August 21, 2017).

COPE (Community Outreach and Patient Empowerment) Program. 2017. *NB3 Water First Initiative with the COPE Program.* https://www.youtube.com/watch?v=F1ULSvw0RnI&feature=youtu.be (accessed August 23, 2017).

Council on Environmental Health. 2016. Prevention of childhood lead toxicity. *Pediatrics* 138(1):e20161493.

Cradock, A. L., J. L. Barrett, E. L. Kenney, C. M. Giles, Z. J. Ward, M. W. Long, S. C. Resch, A. A. Pipito, E. R. Wei, and S. L. Gortmaker. 2017. Using cost-effectiveness analysis to prioritize policy and programmatic approaches to physical activity promotion and obesity prevention in childhood. *Preventive Medicine* 95(Suppl):S17–S27.

de Ruyter, J. C., M. R. Olthof, J. C. Seidell, and M. B. Katan. 2012. A trial of sugar-free or sugar-sweetened beverages and body weight in children. *New England Journal of Medicine* 367(15):1397–1406.

Dietz, W. H., and S. L. Gortmaker. 2016. New strategies to prioritize nutrition, physical activity, and obesity interventions. *American Journal of Preventive Medicine* 51(5):e145–e150.

Drewnowski, A., C. D. Rehm, and F. Constant. 2013. Water and beverage consumption among children age 4-13y in the United States: Analyses of 2005–2010 NHANES data. *Nutrition Journal* 12:85.

Edwards, M., S. Triantafyllidou, and D. Best. 2009. Elevated blood lead in young children due to lead-contaminated drinking water: Washington, DC, 2001–2004. *Environmental Science and Technology* 43(5):1618–1623.

Falbe, J., H. R. Thompson, C. M. Becker, N. Rojas, C. E. McCulloch, and K. A. Madsen. 2016. Impact of the Berkeley excise tax on sugar-sweetened beverage consumption. *American Journal of Public Health* 106(10):1865–1871.

Food Service Guidelines Federal Workgroup. 2017. *Food service guidelines for federal facilities*. Washington, DC: U.S. Department of Health and Human Services.

Garasky, S., K. Mbwana, A. Romualdo, A. Tenaglio, and M. Roy. 2016. *Foods typically purchased by SNAP households*. Alexandria, VA: Food and Nutrition Services, U.S. Department of Agriculture.

Giddings, S. S., and J. A. Mennella. 2016. *Has the world become too sweet?* https://professional.heart.org/professional/ScienceNews/UCM_487623_Has-the-World-Become-Too-Sweet.jsp (accessed August 8, 2017).

Goldberg, J. P., S. C. Folta, M. Eliasziw, S. Koch-Weser, C. D. Economos, K. L. Hubbard, L. A. Tanskey, C. M. Wright, and A. Must. 2015. Great taste, less waste: A cluster-randomized trial using a communications campaign to improve the quality of foods brought from home to school by elementary school children. *Preventive Medicine* 74:103–110.

Gortmaker, S. L., Y. C. Wang, M. W. Long, C. M. Giles, Z. J. Ward, J. L. Barrett, E. L. Kenney, K. R. Sonneville, A. S. Afzal, S. C. Resch, and A. L. Cradock. 2015. Three interventions that reduce childhood obesity are projected to save more than they cost to implement. *Health Affairs (Millwood)* 34(11):1932–1939.

Grimes, C. A., E. A. Szymlek-Gay, K. J. Campbell, and T. A. Nicklas. 2015. Food sources of total energy and nutrients among U.S. infants and toddlers: National Health and Nutrition Examination Survey 2005-2012. *Nutrients* 7(8):6797–6836.

Grimes, C. A., E. A. Szymlek-Gay, and T. A. Nicklas. 2017. Beverage consumption among U.S. children aged 0-24 months: National Health and Nutrition Examination Survey (NHANES). *Nutrients* 9(3):E264.

Harris, J. L., and S. K. Graff. 2012. Protecting young people from junk food advertising: Implications of psychological research for first amendment law. *American Journal of Public Health* 102(2):214–222.

Harris, J. L., K. D. Brownell, and J. A. Bargh. 2009. The food marketing defense model: Integrating psychological research to protect youth and inform public policy. *Social Issues Policy Review* 3(1):211–271.

Harris, J. L., M. B. Schwartz, M. LoDolce, C. Munsell, F. Fleming-Milici, J. Elsey, S. Liu, M. Hyary, R. Gross, C. Hazen, and C. Dembek. 2014. *Sugary drink FACTS 2014: Some progress but much room for improvement in marketing to youth*. http://www.sugarydrinkfacts.org/resources/sugarydrinkfacts_report.pdf (accessed September 6, 2017).

Heyman, M. B., and S. A. Abrams. 2017. Fruit juice in infants, children, and adolescents: Current recommendations. *Pediatrics* 139(6):e20170967.

HHS/USDA (U.S. Department of Health and Human Services/U.S. Department of Agriculture). 2015a. *Dietary Guidelines for Americans 2015-2020: Eighth edition*. https://health.gov/dietaryguidelines/2015/guidelines (accessed August 18, 2017).

HHS/USDA. 2015b. *Scientific report of the 2015 Dietary Guidelines Advisory Committee*. Washington, DC: Agricultural Research Services, U.S. Department of Agriculture.

Horizon Foundation. 2014. *Better beverage finder*. http://www.betterbeveragefinder.org (accessed August 23, 2017).

IOM (Institute of Medicine). 2006. *Food marketing to children and youth: Threat or opportunity?* Washington, DC: The National Academies Press.

Kant, A. K., and B. I. Graubard. 2010. Contributors of water intake in U.S. children and adolescents: Associations with dietary and meal characteristics—National Health and Nutrition Examination Survey 2005–2006. *American Journal of Clinical Nutrition* 92(4): 887–896.

Katan, M. B., J. C. de Ruyter, L. D. Kuijper, C. C. Chow, K. D. Hall, and M. R. Olthof. 2016. Impact of masked replacement of sugar-sweetened with sugar-free beverages on body weight increases with initial BMI: Secondary analysis of data from an 18 month double-blind trial in children. *PLoS ONE* 11(7):e0159771.

Kelly, B., M. L. King, K. Chapman, E. Boyland, A. E. Bauman, and L. A. Baur. 2015. A hierarchy of unhealthy food promotion effects: Identifying methodological approaches and knowledge gaps. *American Journal of Public Health* 105(4):e86–e95.

Kenney, E. L., S. L. Gortmaker, J. E. Carter, M. C. Howe, J. F. Reiner, and A. L. Cradock. 2015a. Grab a cup, fill it up! An intervention to promote the convenience of drinking water and increase student water consumption during school lunch. *American Journal of Public Health* 105(9):1777–1783.

Kenney, E. L., M. W. Long, A. L. Cradock, and S. L. Gortmaker. 2015b. Prevalence of inadequate hydration among U.S. children and disparities by gender and race/ethnicity: National Health and Nutrition Examination Survey, 2009–2012. *American Journal of Public Health* 105(8):e113–e118.

Long, M. W., Z. J. Ward, J. L. Barrett, A. L. Cradock, S. C. Resch, Y. C. Wang, C. M. Giles, and S. L. Gortmaker. 2016. *Taxing sugar-sweetened beverages estimated to reduce racial/ethnic disparities in U.S. obesity prevalence.* Paper presented at American Public Health Association 2016 Annual Meeting and Expo.

Ludwig, D. S., K. E. Peterson, and S. L. Gortmaker. 2001. Relation between consumption of sugar-sweetened drinks and childhood obesity: A prospective, observational analysis. *Lancet* 357(9255):505–508.

May, L., C. Borger, N. Weinfield, C. MacAllum, J. DeMatteis, S. McNutt, S. Whaley, L. Ritchie, and L. Sallack. 2017. *WIC Infant and Toddler Feeding Practices Study–2: Infant year report.* Rockville, MD: Westat.

Miles, G., and A. M. Siega-Riz. 2017. Trends in food and beverage consumption among infants and toddlers: 2005-2012. *Pediatrics* 139(6):e20163290.

Mozaffarian, D., T. Hao, E. B. Rimm, W. C. Willett, and F. B. Hu. 2011. Changes in diet and lifestyle and long-term weight gain in women and men. *New England Journal of Medicine* 364(25):2392–2404.

Muckelbauer, R., L. Libuda, K. Clausen, A. M. Toschke, T. Reinehr, and M. Kersting. 2009. Promotion and provision of drinking water in schools for overweight prevention: Randomized, controlled cluster trial. *Pediatrics* 123(4):e661–e667.

Munsell, C. R., J. L. Harris, V. Sarda, and M. B. Schwartz. 2016. Parents' beliefs about the healthfulness of sugary drink options: Opportunities to address misperceptions. *Public Health Nutrition* 19(1):46–54.

NASEM (National Academies of Sciences, Engineering, and Medicine). 2017. *Strategies to limit sugar-sweetened beverage consumption in young children: Proceedings of a workshop—in brief.* Washington, DC: The National Academies Press.

NCCOR (National Collaborative on Childhood Obesity Research). 2016. *SNAP-Ed.* http://www.nccor.org/nccor-tools/snap-ed-toolkit (accessed August 21, 2017).

Nemours Foundation. 2017. *Let's move! child care.* https://healthykidshealthyfuture.org (accessed August 21, 2017).

NICHQ (National Initiative for Children's Health Quality). 2013. *Next steps: A practitioner's guide for themed follow-up visits for their patients to achieve a healthy weight.* Elk Grove Village, IL: American Academy of Pediatrics.

Ogden, C. L., B. K. Kit, M. D. Carroll, and S. Park. 2011. Consumption of sugar drinks in the United States, 2005-2008. *NCHS Data Brief* (71):1–8.

Ogden, C. L., M. D. Carroll, B. K. Kit, and K. M. Flegal. 2012. Prevalence of obesity and trends in body mass index among U.S. children and adolescents, 1999–2010. *JAMA* 307(5):483–490.

Oliveira, V. 2017. *The food assistance landscape: FY 2016 Annual Report, EIB-169*. Washington, DC: Economic Research Service, U.S. Department of Agriculture.

Patel, A. I., D. J. Shapiro, Y. C. Wang, and M. D. Cabana. 2013. Sociodemographic characteristics and beverage intake of children who drink tap water. *American Journal of Preventive Medicine* 45(1):75–82.

Peters, J., J. Beck, J. Lande, X. Pan, M. Cardel, K. Ayoob, and J. O. Hill. 2016. Using healthy defaults in Walt Disney World restuarants to improve nutritional choices. *Journal of the Association for Consumer Research* 1(1):92–103.

Piernas, C., S. W. Ng, M. A. Mendez, P. Gordon-Larsen, and B. M. Popkin. 2015. A dynamic panel model of the associations of sweetened beverage purchases with dietary quality and food-purchasing patterns. *American Journal of Epidemiology* 181(9):661–671.

Pomeranz, J. L. 2010. Television food marketing to children revisited: The Federal Trade Commission has the constitutional and statutory authority to regulate. *Journal of Law, Medicine, and Ethics* 38(1):98–116.

President and Fellows of Harvard College. 2015. *CHOICES (Childhood Obesity Intervention Cost Effectiveness Study)*. http://choicesproject.org (accessed August 15, 2017).

Public Health Advocates. 2017. *Kick the can*. http://www.kickthecan.info (accessed September 5, 2017).

Public Health Law Center. 2017. *Healthy eating, active play, screen time best practices*. http://www.publichealthlawcenter.org/heal/ChildCareMaps.html (accessed August 22, 2017).

Raynor, H. A., K. M. Osterholt, C. N. Hart, E. Jelalian, P. Vivier, and R. R. Wing. 2012. Efficacy of U.S. paediatric obesity primary care guidelines: Two randomized trials. *Pediatric Obesity* 7(1):28–38.

Ritchie, L., J. Rausa, A. Patel, E. Baraff-Guajardo, and K. Hecht. 2012. *Providing water with meals is not a concern for young children: Summary of the literature and best practice recommendations*. Oakland: California Food Policy Advocates.

Roberto, C. A., D. Wong, A. Musicus, and D. Hammond. 2016. The influence of sugar-sweetened beverage health warning labels on parents' choices. *Pediatrics* 137(2):e20153185.

Rosinger, A., K. Herrick, J. Gahche, and S. Park. 2017. Sugar-sweetened beverage consumption among U.S. youth, 2011–2014. *NCHS Data Brief* (271):1–8.

Schwartz, M. B., K. E. Henderson, M. Read, and T. Cornelius. 2017. Student acceptance of plain milk increases significantly 2 years after flavored milk is removed from school cafeterias: An observational study. *Journal of the Academy of Nutritrition and Dietetics* S2212–S2672(17):30550–30556.

Silver, L. 2017. *Jobs, revenue rise after Berkeley soda tax*. http://www.phi.org/resources/?resource=berkeley-soda-tax-boosts-jobs-revenues (accessed September 5, 2017).

Silver, L. D., S. W. Ng, S. Ryan-Ibarra, L. S. Taillie, M. Induni, D. R. Miles, J. M. Poti, and B. M. Popkin. 2017. Changes in prices, sales, consumer spending, and beverage consumption one year after a tax on sugar-sweetened beverages in Berkeley, California, U.S.: A before-and-after study. *PLoS Medicine* 14(4):e1002283.

Solomon, R. C., and F. Flores. 2001. *Building trust: In business, politics, relationships, and life*. New York: Oxford University Press.

Sonneville, K. R., M. W. Long, S. L. Rifas-Shiman, K. Kleinman, M. W. Gillman, and E. M. Taveras. 2015. Juice and water intake in infancy and later beverage intake and adiposity: Could juice be a gateway drink? *Obesity (Silver Spring)* 23(1):170–176.

Triantafyllidou, S., and M. Edwards. 2012. Lead (Pb) in tap water and in blood: Implications for lead exposure in the United States. *Critical Reviews in Environmental Science and Techonology* 42(13):1297–1352.

UNC (University of North Carolina) at Chapel Hill. 2017. *Go NAP SACC!* https://gonapsacc.org (accessed August 21, 2017).

VanEpps, E. M., and C. A. Roberto. 2016. The influence of sugar-sweetened beverage warnings: A randomized trial of adolescents' choices and beliefs. *American Journal of Preventive Medicine* 51(5):664–672.

Wang, Y. C., S. N. Bleich, and S. L. Gortmaker. 2008. Increasing caloric contribution from sugar-sweetened beverages and 100% fruit juices among U.S. children and adolescents, 1988-2004. *Pediatrics.* 121(6):e1604–e1614.

Wang, Y. C., P. Coxson, Y. M. Shen, L. Goldman, and K. Bibbins-Domingo. 2012. A penny-per-ounce tax on sugar-sweetened beverages would cut health and cost burdens of diabetes. *Health Affairs (Millwood)* 31(1):199–207.

Watowicz, R. P., S. E. Anderson, G. L. Kaye, and C. A. Taylor. 2015. Energy contribution of beverages in U.S. children by age, weight, and consumer status. *Childhood Obesity* 11(4):475–483.

WCRF (World Cancer Research Fund). 2015. *Curbing global sugar consumption: Effective food policy actions to help promote healthy diets and tackle obesity.* London, UK: World Cancer Research Fund International.

Wescott, R. F., B. M. Fitzpatrick, and E. Phillips. 2012. Industry self-regulation to improve student health: Quantifying changes in beverage shipments to schools. *American Journal of Public Health* 102(10):1928–1935.

WHO (World Health Organization). 2015. *Guideline: Sugar intake for adults and children.* Geneva, Switzerland: WHO Press.

Wilcox, B. L., D. Kunkel, J. Cantor, P. Dowrick, S. Linn, and E. Palmer. 2004. *APA task force on advertising and children.* Washington, DC: American Psychological Association.

Wright, D. R., E. L. Kenney, C. M. Giles, M. W. Long, Z. J. Ward, S. C. Resch, M. L. Moodie, R. C. Carter, Y. C. Wang, G. Sacks, B. A. Swinburn, S. L. Gortmaker, and A. L. Cradock. 2015. Modeling the cost effectiveness of child care policy changes in the U.S. *American Journal of Preventive Medicine* 49(1):135–147.

Zheng, M., A. Rangan, N. J. Olsen, L. B. Andersen, N. Wedderkopp, P. Kristensen, A. Grontved, M. Ried-Larsen, S. M. Lempert, M. Allman-Farinelli, and B. L. Heitmann. 2015. Substituting sugar-sweetened beverages with water or milk is inversely associated with body fatness development from childhood to adolescence. *Nutrition* 31(1):38–44.

Appendix A

Workshop Agenda

A Workshop on Strategies to Limit Sugar-Sweetened Beverage Consumption in Young Children: Evaluation of Federal, State, and Local Policies and Programs

National Academy of Sciences Building
2101 Constitution Avenue, NW
Room 125
Washington, DC 20418

WORKSHOP OBJECTIVES

- Provide an overview of current and emerging strategies to reduce consumption of sugar-sweetened beverages by young children from 0 to 5 years of age and explore the evidence on effectiveness.
- Contextualize the strategies by considering patterns and trends in beverage consumption broadly, and sugar-sweetened beverage consumption specifically, in U.S. children.
- Examine current guidelines for beverage intake applicable to children 5 years of age and younger.
- Explore the role of industry in sugar-sweetened beverage intake in young children.
- Identify where knowledge gaps and opportunities exist to inform future policies, programs, and strategies.

AGENDA

WEDNESDAY, JUNE 21, 2017

7:30 AM **Registration Opens**

8:00 **Welcome**
Karen Weber Cullen, Baylor College of Medicine, Planning Committee Chair

8:10 **Sponsors' Opening Remarks** (5 minutes each)
Tina Kauh, Robert Wood Johnson Foundation
Judi Larsen, The California Endowment (remote)
Robert Post, Chobani Foundation

SESSION I: Setting the Stage

Session Objectives:

- *To explore the current prevalence and trends in beverage intake among young children*
- *To understand where disparities in sugar-sweetened beverage intake exist*
- *To consider how young children's intake could change if sugar-sweetened beverages are reduced or eliminated from their diets*

8:25 **Session Overview**
Moderator: Leann Birch, University of Georgia

8:35 **Prevalence, Trends, and Disparities in Beverage Consumption Among Young Children 0–24 Months from NHANES**
Anna Maria Siega-Riz, University of Virginia School of Medicine

8:45 **Prevalence, Trends, and Disparities in Beverage Consumption Among Young Children 0 to 4 years of Age: Findings from FITS 2016**
Mary Story, Duke University

9:10	**Cost-Effective Strategies to Limit Sugar-Sweetened Beverages in Children: What Can We Expect?** *Steven Gortmaker, Harvard T.H. Chan School of Public Health*
9:35	**Drinking Water: What Do We Need to Know and Do?** *Christina Hecht, University of California Nutrition Policy Institute*
10:00	**Facilitated Discussion with Audience** *Session Speakers*
10:35	**Break**

SESSION II: Guidelines for Beverage Intake Applicable to Children 5 Years and Younger

Session Objectives:

- *To review prominent guidelines that offer guidance on beverage intake of young children*
- *To understand the evidence inputs that were used to develop the guidelines*
- *To explore any differences or gaps that currently exist across guidelines*

10:50	**Session Overview** *Moderator: Esa Davis, University of Pittsburgh*
10:55	**Scientific Report of the 2015 Dietary Guidelines Advisory Committee, Beverage Recommendations: Sugar-Sweetened Beverages and Water** *Rafael Pérez-Escamilla, Yale University*
11:20	**AAP Guidelines Regarding Sugar-Sweetened Beverages for Children Younger Than 5 Years of Age** *Stephen Daniels, University of Colorado School of Medicine*
11:45	**Facilitated Discussion with Audience** *Session Speakers*
12:00 PM	**Break for Lunch**

SESSION III: An Exploration of Federal, State, and Local Policies and Programs: Opportunities and Challenges to Influence Beverage Consumption in Young Children

Session Objectives:

- *To provide an overview of policies, programs, and practices at the federal, state, and local levels that affect beverage consumption in a large segment of the population, especially in children 0 to 5 years of age*
- *To understand the scope of the policies, programs, and regulations and the population groups who are and who are not affected or served*
- *To discuss evidence that justifies implementation and approaches to monitoring effectiveness, particularly related to beverage consumption*

1:00 **Session Overview**
Moderator: Christina Economos, Tufts University

1:05 **Regulations and Policies for Beverages in Federal Nutrition Programs**
Sara Bleich, Harvard T.H. Chan School of Public Health

1:20 **State and Local Public Health Opportunities to Support Healthy Beverage Intake Among Children 0 to 5 Years**
Heidi Blanck, Centers for Disease Control and Prevention

1:35 **State-Level Policies in the Child Care Setting**
Natasha Frost, Public Health Law Center

1:50 **A Local Perspective: New York City's Strategies to Reduce Sugary Drink Consumption**
Kim Kessler, New York City Department of Health and Mental Hygiene

2:05 **Facilitated Discussion with Audience**
Session Speakers

2:30 **Break**

SESSION IV: Innovations and Challenges of Emerging Strategies

Session Objectives:

- *To explore novel interventions crossing various sectors that could potentially be scaled up*
- *To discuss strategies to evaluate innovative and emerging policies, programs, and approaches*

2:40 **Session Overview**
Moderator: Tracy Fox, Food, Nutrition and Policy Consultants, LLC

2:45 **COPE Water First! Initiative with NB3 Foundation**
Henrietta Sandoval-Soland, COPE Project

3:05 **Howard County Unsweetened: Policy + Outreach + Media = Change**
Marlene Schwartz, Rudd Center for Food Policy and Obesity

3:25 **Facilitated Discussion with Audience**
Henrietta Sandoval-Soland and Marlene Schwartz

3:40 **Local Ordinances and Regulations: Feasibility, Challenges, and Impact**
Moderator: Anna Maria Siega-Riz, University of Virginia School of Medicine
Panelists: *Margo Wootan, Center for Science in the Public Interest*
Lynn Silver, Public Health Institute
Michelle Mello, Stanford Law School

4:35 **Facilitated Discussion with Audience**
Panelists

4:55 **Reflections on the Day**
Karen Weber Cullen, Baylor College of Medicine, Planning Committee Chair

5:00 **Adjourn First Day**

THURSDAY, JUNE 22, 2017

7:30 AM	**Registration Opens**
8:00	**Summary of Day 1 and Overview of Day 2** *Karen Weber Cullen, Baylor College of Medicine, Planning Committee Chair*

SESSION V: The Role of Industry in Sugar-Sweetened Beverage Consumption

Session Objectives:

- *To consider industry's role in the current consumption patterns in the United States, particularly among young children*
- *To explore strategies for industry to improve children's health by reducing sugar-sweetened beverages through approaches such as marketing, partnerships, and product reformulation*

8:10	**Session Overview** *Moderator: Barbara Devaney, Mathematica Policy Research*
8:15	**Marketing Sugary Drinks to Young Children ... and Their Parents** *Jennifer Harris, Rudd Center for Food Policy and Obesity*
8:40	**Sugar-Sweetened Beverages: Voluntary and Regulatory Industry Approaches** *Richard Black, Quadrant D Consulting*
9:00	**Partnerships with Industry to Improve Beverage Choices of Young Children** *Anne Ferree, Alliance for a Healthier Generation*
9:20	**Facilitated Discussion with Audience** *Session Speakers*
10:00	**Break**

SESSION VI: Reflections, Gaps, and Opportunities

Session Objectives:

- *To reflect upon and summarize key messages from the preceding sessions*
- *To explore the evidence gaps and research needs that exist*
- *To consider opportunities to fill gaps*

10:20 **Session Overview**
Karen Weber Cullen, Baylor College of Medicine, Planning Committee Chair

10:25 **A Summary of the Workshop Presentations**
Virginia Stallings, Children's Healthcare of Philadelphia

10:45 **Panel Discussion**
Moderator: Virginia Stallings, Children's Healthcare of Philadelphia
Panelists: *Richard Black, Quadrant D Consulting*
Stephen Daniels, University of Colorado School of Medicine
Marlene Schwartz, Rudd Center for Food Policy and Obesity
Mary Story, Duke University

11:25 **Facilitated Discussion with Audience**
Panelists

11:45 **Wrap-Up and Reflections on the Workshop**
Karen Weber Cullen, Baylor College of Medicine, Planning Committee Chair

12:00 PM Adjourn Workshop

Appendix B

Speaker and Moderator Biographical Sketches

Leann Birch, Ph.D., is the William P. "Bill" Flatt professor in the Department of Foods and Nutrition at the University of Georgia. As a developmental psychologist, her research career has focused on individual and contextual factors that influence the developing controls of food intake and obesity risk among infants, children, and adolescents. Early research from Dr. Birch's laboratory on factors affecting the developing controls of food intake in the first years of life, including food preferences and responsiveness to portion size and energy density, have contributed to the evidence base on behavioral factors implicated in the development of childhood obesity. These findings laid the groundwork for exploring individual, familial, and contextual factors that shape the development of differences in eating behavior and obesity. This research has informed randomized controlled trials designed to affect maternal caregiving and infant feeding and sleeping to prevent obesity beginning in infancy. She is the author of more than 200 publications and internationally recognized for her research.

Richard Black, Ph.D., is a principal at Quadrant D Consulting and most recently served as vice president of Global Nutrition Sciences PepsiCo, where he led the development of a nutrition strategy that fueled PepsiCo's innovation and portfolio transformation through nutrition science. Prior to joining PepsiCo, Dr. Black worked for Mondeléz International, where he served as vice president, Nutrition, and chief nutrition officer. Dr. Black brings a wealth of leadership and technical expertise from the consumer packaged and pharmaceutical industries. In his 25-year career, Dr. Black has also held nutrition and health and wellness leadership positions at Nestlé, Kellogg's,

Novartis, and Kraft with a focus on carbohydrate, dairy, sports nutrition, micro/macro ingredients and gut health/microbiome. In addition, Dr. Black was an assistant professor at the University of Toronto, Department of Nutrition Sciences, and he currently is an adjunct professor of the practice at the Friedman School of Nutrition Science and Policy at Tufts University. Dr. Black also served on Health Canada advisory panels, developing policies on health claims and addition of micronutrients in food. He holds his Ph.D. in psychology of eating behavior and has two B.S. degrees, one in chemistry and the other in psychology, both from McMaster University.

Captain Heidi Blanck, Ph.D., is the chief of the Obesity Prevention and Control Branch at the Centers for Disease Control and Prevention (CDC) in the Division of Nutrition, Physical Activity, and Obesity. She has more than 18 years of CDC experience as a public health epidemiologist and has authored more than 100 manuscripts. Dr. Blanck oversees CDC's monitoring of state obesity prevalence and key supports for healthy eating and active living. Staff within the branch focus on providing surveillance, applied research, guidelines development, and technical assistance to state, territorial, tribal, and local health agencies. Topics include food service guidelines, healthy weight programs for children, food insecurity, body mass index, and chronic disease factors, including fruits and vegetables, drinking water, added sugars, and sugar-sweetened beverages. Her work focuses on changes in environments across multiple settings (i.e., early care and education, medical care, worksites) with an emphasis on ensuring all communities have a fair chance at health. She is senior advisor to CDC's extramural Nutrition and Obesity Policy Research and Evaluation Network (NOPREN) and the National Collaborative on Childhood Obesity Research (NCCOR). Dr. Blanck received her Ph.D. from Emory University, where she is an adjunct professor. She also serves as a member of the National Academies of Sciences, Engineering, and Medicine's Roundtable on Obesity Solutions.

Sara Bleich, Ph.D., is a professor of public health policy at the Harvard T.H. Chan School of Public Health in the Department of Health Policy and Management. She is also the Carol K. Pforzheimer professor at the Radcliffe Institute for Advanced Study. Dr. Bleich's scholarship lies at the nexus of health policy and health services research. Her research provides evidence to support policy alternatives for obesity prevention and control, particularly among populations at higher risk for obesity. This work is composed of three complementary streams of inquiry: (1) pathways for change in major drivers of calorie intake, (2) health provider opportunities to improve obesity care, and (3) novel environmental strategies for obesity prevention. A signature theme throughout her work is an interest in asking simple, meaningful questions about the complex problem of obesity, which can fill important gaps in the literature. Her research has been published in journals such as the *New England Journal of Medicine*, *Health Affairs*, and the *American Journal of Public Health*, and she has been featured in outlets such as *The New York Times*, *The Wall Street Journal*, and National Public Radio. Dr. Bleich is the past recipient of an award for "most outstanding abstract" at the International Conference on Obesity in Sydney, Australia, an award for "best research manuscript" in the journal *Obesity*, and an award for excellence in public interest communication from the Frank Conference. Dr. Bleich was recently appointed as a White House Fellow (2015–2016) where she was a senior policy advisor to the U.S. Department of Agriculture and the First Lady's Let's Move initiative. She holds degrees from Columbia (B.A., psychology) and Harvard (Ph.D., health policy).

Karen Weber Cullen, Dr.P.H., R.D., is a professor of pediatrics-nutrition at the U.S. Department of Agriculture, Agricultural Research Services (USDA-ARS) Children's Nutrition Research Center, Baylor College of Medicine. Her primary research interest is prevention of obesity and diet-related chronic diseases. Her current research includes evaluating the effect of the new Child and Adult Care Food Program (CACFP) meal guidelines on child consumption and costs and examining the contribution of school meals to children's daily dietary intake. Dr. Cullen previously served as a member of the Institute of Medicine's (IOM's) Committee on Nutrition Standards for National School Lunch and Breakfast Programs and the Committee to Review Child and Adult Care Food Program Meal Requirements. She was also a member of the IOM Planning Committee on the Review of the Child and Adult Care Food Program Meal Requirements: A Workshop, and chair of the Planning Committee for the Workshop on National Nutrition Education Curriculum Standards, held on March 11–12, 2014. Dr. Cullen's professional memberships include the American Dietetic Association and the Texas Dietetic Association (Distinguished Scientist Award in 2001). Dr. Cullen has an M.S. in nutrition from Case Western Reserve University and a Dr.P.H. in health promotion and health education from The University of Texas School of Public Health.

Stephen R. Daniels, M.D., Ph.D., FAAP, held numerous academic and clinical appointments at the University of Cincinnati College of Medicine and Cincinnati Children's Hospital before joining the University of Colorado School of Medicine in 2006 as professor and the chair of the Department of Pediatrics. Dr. Daniels is also pediatrician-in-chief and L. Joseph Butterfield chair in pediatrics at Children's Hospital Colorado. He received his M.D. from the University of Chicago, his M.P.H. from Harvard University, and his Ph.D. in Epidemiology from the University of North Carolina. Dr. Daniels's area of expertise is preventive cardiology, with a longtime interest in the application of sophisticated epidemiologic and biostatistical methods to pediatric clinical research problems. His studies have focused on better understanding the causes of blood pressure elevation and cholesterol abnormalities in children and adolescents, particularly the role that obesity may play in these health issues. He has also researched the development of structural and functional abnormalities in the heart and vascular system, including cardiovascular abnormalities occurring in pediatric patients with diabetes mellitus, as well as the relationship of left ventricular hypertrophy to obesity and hypertension. The role of lifestyle factors, such as diet and physical activity, is central to many of Dr. Daniels's studies. Dr. Daniels has served as associate editor for the *Journal of Pediatrics* since 1995. He is co-author of *Medical Epidemiology*, an introductory textbook for medical students, and co-author and editor of the book *Pediatric Prevention of Atherosclerotic Cardiovascular Disease*. In 2015, he was awarded the Gold Heart Award by the American Heart Association (AHA), which is the AHA's highest volunteer honor.

Esa Matius Davis, M.D., M.P.H., FAAFP, is a National of Institutes of Health (NIH) funded clinical researcher with a patient-oriented research program focused on obesity-related maternal and child health outcomes and in comparative effectiveness research in obesity and tobacco. Much of her work has focused on understanding the development of obesity in women. She specifically contributed to the field by investigating the perinatal, cultural, and behavioral factors associated with the racial and socioeconomic disparities in obesity among women that have persisted for decades. She published a novel conceptual framework that has been highly cited to help guide the testing of hypotheses associated with weight change during pregnancy and the long-term development of obesity and related disparities. Dr. Davis has contributed new analytic methods in investigating pregnancy factors associated with the development of maternal obesity and related outcomes. She is currently the principal investigator of an NIH-funded randomized controlled trial titled "Comparison of Two Screening Strategies for Gestational Diabetes, GDM2 Study," which aims to examine differences in perinatal outcomes of women randomized to two screening/diagnostic strategies for gestational diabetes. She has also conducted studies that investigate the association between obesity and cardiac recovery and remodeling in women with postpartum cardiomyopathy. She has served on two Institute of Medicine committees: Implementation and Dissemination of the Pregnancy Weight Gain Guidelines and the Epigenetics and Childhood Obesity. Dr. Davis's research also focuses on reducing risk factors such as hypertension, obesity, smoking, and patient attitudes associated with cardiovascular disease. She is currently a co-investigator on three NIH/U.S. Food and Drug Administration funded randomized controlled trials that are investigating effective strategies for treating hospitalized smokers and evaluating new nicotine standards for cigarettes.

Barbara Devaney, Ph.D., is a nationally recognized expert in maternal and child health, nutrition, and risk-reduction programs for youth. She has played a leading role in many of Mathematica's studies of family formation, children's nutrition, and public health programs. Dr. Devaney codirected Mathematica's Building Strong Families study and served as principal investigator for the firm's evaluation of abstinence education programs, which received the 2009 Outstanding Evaluation Award from the American Evaluation Association. She also oversaw Mathematica's 2002 Feeding Infants and Toddlers Study, which provided detailed information on the food and nutrient intakes of U.S. infants and toddlers. Other evaluations in which she has played a key role have focused on the school lunch and breakfast programs; the Special Supplemental Nutrition Program for Women, Infants, and Children (WIC); and the Food Stamp Program. A long-term employee of the firm, she was previously an assistant professor at Duke University and the Johns Hopkins University. Dr. Devaney has served on scientific committees convened by the National Academies of Sciences, Engineering, and Medicine, and on the policy council of the Association for Public Policy Analysis and Management. She has published widely in peer-reviewed journals, including the *Journal of Policy Analysis and Management*, *American Journal of Clinical Nutrition*, *Journal of the American Dietetic Association*, and the *American Journal of Public Health*. She also presents findings at conferences of researchers, policy makers, and practitioners. She has a Ph.D. in economics from the University of Michigan.

Christina Economos, Ph.D., is a professor and the New Balance chair in childhood nutrition at the Friedman School of Nutrition Science and Policy and Medical School at Tufts University. She is also the co-founder and director of ChildObesity180, a unique organization that brings together leaders from diverse disciplines to generate urgency and find solutions to the childhood obesity epidemic. ChildObesity180 merges the best in nutrition and public health research and practice with the expertise and experience of business, government, and nonprofit leaders. When these perspectives come together, a creative tension exists that balances the academic focus on discovering what works and why, with the entrepreneurial perspective that quick action is needed. As the principal investigator of large-scale research studies, Dr. Economos's goal is to inspire behavior, policy, and environmental change to reduce obesity and improve the health of America's children. She has authored more than 120 scientific publications. At ChildObesity180 she develops, implements, evaluates, and scales up high-impact obesity prevention initiatives. She led the Shape Up Somerville study demonstrating that it is possible to reduce excess weight gain in children through multiple leverage points within an entire community. Dr. Economos's Live Well study was a preventive intervention developed with active input from community partners to moderate or reduce weight gain among new immigrant women and their children. In partnership with Save the Children, she led the CHANGE study, which was designed to improve physical activity and nutrition behaviors in rural communities. Dr. Economos is involved in national obesity and public health activities and has served on four National Academies of Sciences, Engineering, and Medicine committees, including the Roundtable on Obesity Solutions and the Committee on an Evidence Framework for Obesity Prevention Decision Making. In addition, she serves on the American Heart Association's Nutrition Council on Lifestyle and Cardiometabolic Health. Dr. Economos received a B.S. from Boston University, an M.S. in applied physiology and nutrition from Columbia University, and a Ph.D. in nutritional biochemistry from Tufts University.

Anne Ferree, M.P.P., leads the Alliance for a Healthier Generation's engagement with the business sector as part of a multi-faceted approach to ensure environments surrounding children and families promote and provide for good health. She leads a team responsible for negotiating, implementing, and evaluating voluntary agreements with companies, and creating and strengthening partnerships with other nonprofit organizations and government agencies. Ms. Ferree served as the founding leader of the Alliance's Healthy Out-of-School Time initiative, guiding a team of national and field staff to support out-of-school time professionals to create healthier environments for kids. She also led the development of multi-year national agreements with the Boys & Girls Clubs of America and the National Recreation and Park Association. With more than 30 years of experience, Ms. Ferree's career spans private, public, and nonprofit realms. Prior to joining the Alliance, she was a senior leader of the consulting practice of a global architecture, design and planning firm, focused on multi-disciplined approaches to solving complex problems facing counties, cities, and school districts. Ms. Ferree holds a B.S. from Cornell University and an M.P.P. from the University of Southern California.

Tracy Fox, M.P.H., R.D., has more than 25 years of experience working at the federal, state, and local/community levels and with the private sector, with extensive experience in nutrition policy, legislative and regulatory processes, and advocacy. Past and current clients include the U.S. Department of Agriculture, Centers for Disease Control and Prevention, Robert Wood Johnson Foundation, American Heart Association, American Cancer Society, Partnership for a Healthier America, National Head Start, Nemours, grocery stores, and public relations firms. Areas of specialty include child nutrition and health, nutrition education, food insecurity, early care and education, food labeling, and marketing. Ms. Fox is past President of the Society for Nutrition Education and Behavior and has served on the Institute of Medicine's School Foods, Childhood Obesity Prevention Actions for Local Governments, and Front-of-Pack Labeling committees; Feeding America Nutrition Advisory Board; Hannaford Scientific Advisory Board; Montgomery County School Health Council and PTA, Boys and Girls Club of Culver, United Way of Marshall county, Max's Playhouse Daycare, co-manager, Culver Farmers' Market, and Wellness Consultant, Culver Academies. Ms. Fox is a retired commander in the U.S. Navy Reserves.

Natasha Frost, J.D., is a senior staff attorney at the Public Health Law Center. She provides legal technical assistance to nonprofits and stakeholders around the country in developing effective policies to promote healthy eating and active living. Ms. Frost has done extensive research on healthy food and active play in the early care and education setting, including analyzing each state's child care licensing structure and developing several state-specific resources. She also has worked with community members to assess policy opportunities to increase access to healthy, affordable food at the local level. Ms. Frost brings real-world experience into the food system and child care work as an owner of a small restaurant in southern Minnesota, which is currently catering food for a child care center and using the Child and Adult Care Food Program (CACFP) meal pattern standards that will go into effect in 2017. Throughout all her work, Ms. Frost seeks to identify how policies and systems impact health inequities, and how law can be used as a tool for change. Prior to joining the Center, Ms. Frost spent 10 years at the Alliance for Children's Rights, a nonprofit in Los Angeles, California. As the benefits program director, she created and managed a program that represents children and their caregivers to obtain public benefits. She handled more than 300 administrative fair hearings and recovered more than $7,000,000 in funding on behalf of needy children. She also provided consulting and technical support to systemic efforts, including litigation and legislation, designed to overcome barriers to accessing benefits and services.

Steven Gortmaker, Ph.D., is currently a professor of the practice of health sociology at the Harvard T.H. Chan School of Public Health. He directs the Harvard T.H. Chan School of Public Health Prevention Research Center (HPRC), whose mission is to work with community partners to design, implement, and evaluate programs and policies that improve nutrition and physical activity; reduce overweight and chronic disease risk among children, youth, and their families; and to reduce and eliminate disparities in these outcomes. Dr. Gortmaker serves as senior advisor to the Healthy Eating Research Program of the Robert Wood Johnson Foundation. Current activities include continuing implementation, dissemination, and updating the widely disseminated school curriculums: Planet Health and Eat Well and Keep Moving, the afterschool curriculum co-developed with the YMCA of the USA—Food and Fun, and the Out of School Nutrition and Physical Activity Initiative. Current major research includes the CHOICES project funded by the JPB Foundation that is evaluating the cost-effectiveness of more than 40 childhood obesity preventive interventions. Dr. Gortmaker has been an author and co-author of more than 210 published research articles, including the first report in the United States concerning the obesity epidemic among children, the first longitudinal study linking increases in sugar-sweetened beverage intake to increased obesity incidence in youth, the recent four-paper obesity modeling series in the *Lancet*, and recent cost-effectiveness papers in the *American Journal of Preventive Medicine* and *Health Affairs*.

Jennifer Harris, Ph.D., M.B.A., is the director of marketing initiatives at the Rudd Center for Food Policy and Obesity and associate professor in allied health sciences at University of Connecticut. She leads a multidisciplinary team of researchers who study food marketing to children, adolescents, and parents, and how it affects their diets and health. Dr. Harris is a leading expert on food marketing to youth, and her research is widely used by the public health community and policy makers to improve the food marketing environment surrounding children and adolescents in the United States and worldwide. Specific areas of research include monitoring and evaluating the amount, types, and nutrition quality of food and drinks marketed to youth and families; the psychology of food marketing and its effect on health behaviors; and identifying effective policy solutions. Her current research focuses on targeted marketing and health disparities affecting black and Hispanic youth; new forms of marketing targeted to youth on social media and mobile devices; and effects of food marketing on what and how parents feed their babies and young children. Dr. Harris received her B.A. from Northwestern University and M.B.A. in marketing from the Wharton School. Before returning to graduate school, she was a marketing executive for 18 years, including at American Express as a vice president in consumer marketing and as principal in a marketing strategy consulting firm. Dr. Harris completed her Ph.D. in social psychology at Yale University with Dr. John Bargh and Dr. Kelly Brownell.

Christina Hecht, Ph.D., is a senior policy advisor at University of California Nutrition Policy Institute (NPI). Dr. Hecht leads NPI's work in drinking water access and consumption. She coordinates the National Drinking Water Alliance, a network of individuals and organizations across the United States working to ensure that all children in the United States can drink water in the places where they live, learn, and play. Dr. Hecht graduated from Stanford University with a B.A. in human biology, and from the Johns Hopkins School of Hygiene and Public Health with a Ph.D. in population dynamics.

Kim Kessler, J.D., is the assistant commissioner for the Bureau of Chronic Disease Prevention and Tobacco Control at the New York City Department of Health and Mental Hygiene (NYC DOHMH), where she leads an interdisciplinary team focused on promoting healthy behaviors and shaping the local environment to facilitate healthy and active living for all New Yorkers. The Bureau focuses on addressing key risk factors that lead to chronic disease—including poor nutrition, inadequate physical activity, and tobacco use—while also working to leverage clinical tools and settings to promote public health. Prior to joining the Health Department, Ms. Kessler helped to launch the Resnick Program for Food Law and Policy at the University of California, Los Angeles, School of Law. Before that, she served as the food policy coordinator for the City of New York, an appointed position in the Mayor's Office, where she coordinated municipal food policies and initiatives related to improved retail access to nutritious foods, urban agriculture, healthy food procurement, and combating obesity. She received an A.B. degree in political science from Brown University and a J.D. degree, magna cum laude, from the New York University School of Law.

Michelle Mello, J.D., Ph.D., conducts empirical research into issues at the intersection of law, ethics, and health policy. She is the author of more than 160 articles and book chapters on the medical malpractice system, medical errors and patient safety, public health law, research ethics, the obesity epidemic, pharmaceuticals, and other topics. A recipient of a number of awards for her research, she was elected to the National Academy of Medicine at the age of 40. She has served on three National Academies of Sciences, Engineering, and Medicine ad hoc committees. From 2000 to 2014, Dr. Mello was a professor at the Harvard School of Public Health, where she directed the School's Program in Law and Public Health. In 2013–2014 she was a lab fellow at Harvard University's Edmond J. Safra Center for Ethics. Dr. Mello teaches courses in torts and public health law. She holds a J.D. from the Yale Law School, a Ph.D. in Health Policy and Administration from the University of North Carolina at Chapel Hill, an M.Phil. from Oxford University, where she was a Marshall Scholar, and a B.A. from Stanford University.

Rafael Pérez-Escamilla, Ph.D., is a professor of epidemiology and public health, director of the Office of Public Health Practice, and director of the Global Health Concentration at the Yale School of Public Health. His global public health nutrition and food security research program has led to improvements in breastfeeding programs, iron deficiency anemia among infants, household food security measurement and outcomes, and community nutrition education programs. His health disparities research involves assessing the effect of community health workers at improving behavioral and metabolic outcomes among Latinos with type 2 diabetes. He has published more than 200 research articles, two books, and numerous journal supplements, book chapters, and technical reports. He is a member of the Food and Nutrition Board of the National Academies of Sciences, Engineering, and Medicine. He has been a senior advisor to maternal–child nutrition programs as well as household food security measurement projects funded by the World Health Organization; Pan American Health Organization; United Nations International Children's Emergency Fund; Food and Agriculture Organization of the United Nations; United Nations Educational, Scientific and Cultural Organization; United Nations Development Programme; Centers for Disease Control and Prevention; U.S. Department of Agriculture; U.S. Agency for International Development; World Bank; Bill & Melinda Gates Foundation; and the governments of Brazil, Colombia, and Mexico.

Henrietta Sandoval-Soland is a retired magistrate judge and has more than 15 years of experience in law enforcement serving as the first female Native American New Mexico State Police Officer. She assisted in implementing a nonprofit organization in two New Mexico counties that focus on providing support and education to first-time families and their newborn at no cost, and is currently serving a 4-year term as Commissioner with the Navajo Nation Human Rights Commission. Ms. Sandoval-Soland recognizes the importance of multi-cultural differences, traditions, and beliefs in relation to family upbringing and continues to collaborate with other programs and agencies that focus on promoting healthy communities.

Marlene Schwartz, Ph.D., is the director of the Rudd Center for Food Policy and Obesity and professor of human development and family studies at the University of Connecticut. Dr. Schwartz studies how nutrition and wellness policies implemented in child care settings, schools, food banks, and local communities can improve children's health. Dr. Schwartz earned her Ph.D. in psychology from Yale University in 1996. Prior to joining the Rudd Center, she served as co-director of the Yale Center for Eating and Weight Disorders from 1996 to 2006. She has received research grants from the Robert Wood Johnson Foundation, the U.S. Department of Agriculture, and the National Institutes of Health to study the federal food programs, school wellness policies, the effect of food marketing on children, and the relationship between food insecurity and nutrition. In 2014, Dr. Schwartz received the Sarah Samuels Award from the Food and Nutrition Section of the American Public Health Association, and in 2016 she was an honoree at the Connecticut Women's Hall of Fame.

Anna Maria Siega-Riz, Ph.D., is a professor in the departments of public health sciences and obstetrics and gynecology at the University of Virginia School of Medicine. She was previously the associate dean for academic affairs and professor in the departments of epidemiology and nutrition at the Gillings School of Global Public Health, the University of North Carolina (UNC) at Chapel Hill where she still holds an appointment. She has focused her research on maternal nutritional status, including maternal obesity and gestational weight gain and their effect on the short- and long-term outcomes of the mother and child. She studies dietary patterns among Hispanic adults and children. She was a member of the 2015 Dietary Guidelines Advisory Committee; has served on multiple committees for the National Academies of Sciences, Engineering, and Medicine, examining topics from the Special Supplemental Nutrition Program for Women, Infants, and Children food packages to standards for systematic reviews in health care, and recently rotated off the advisory council of the National Heart, Lung, and Blood Institute. She is currently serving on the U.S. Department of Agriculture working group preparing for the dietary guidance during pregnancy for the 2020 report. Dr. Siega-Riz earned a B.S. in public health in nutrition from the UNC at Chapel Hill School of Public Health; an M.S. in food, nutrition, and food service management from UNC at Greensboro; and a Ph.D. in nutrition (minor in epidemiology) from the UNC at Chapel Hill School of Public Health.

Lynn Silver, M.D., M.P.H., is a senior advisor at Public Health Institute (PHI) for chronic disease and obesity and Clinical Professor at the University of California, San Francisco. She works to enhance and strengthen PHI's portfolio of research and programs in chronic diseases, obesity prevention, and global non-communicable diseases. Previously, Dr. Silver served as health officer in Sonoma County, assistant health commissioner in New York City, and as a professor of public health in Brazil for 15 years. In New York City's Department of Health, she led the implementation of forward-thinking strategies to promote population health, including eliminating use of artery-hardening *trans* fats in food establishments—the first such initiative in the nation—and requiring calorie labeling at fast-food restaurants. Dr. Silver received her M.D. and M.P.H. degrees at Johns Hopkins University.

Virginia Stallings, M.D., is a professor of pediatrics at the University of Pennsylvania Perelman School of Medicine, director of the Nutrition Center at the Children's Hospital of Philadelphia, and holds the Jean A. Cortner endowed chair in gastroenterology and nutrition. Dr. Stallings is a pediatrician and a specialist in nutrition and growth in children with chronic illness. Her research interests are in areas of nutrition-related growth and body composition in healthy children and those with chronic disease including obesity, sickle cell disease, osteoporosis, cystic fibrosis, cerebral palsy, Crohn's disease, HIV, and congenital heart disease. She has been extensively involved in pediatric nutrition clinical care and research for more than 25 years. Dr. Stallings plays a broader role in the community of nutrition scientists and physicians as a past or current member of the Institute of Medicine; the National Academies of Sciences, Engineering, and Medicine; and the council of the American Society for Nutrition. She was the chair of the 2007 Institute of Medicine committee report *Nutrition Standards for Foods in Schools: Leading the Way Towards Healthier Youth* and the 2010 committee report *School Meals: Building Blocks for Healthy Children* that led to new policy to improve the nutritional quality of school breakfasts and lunches. Most recently, she chaired the Committee on Food Allergies: Global Burden, Causes, Treatment, Preventions and Public Policy, which published its report *Finding a Path to Safety in Food Allergy: Assessment of the Global Burden, Causes, Prevention, Management, and Public Policy.* She is a former member (1997–2000) and co–vice chair (2000–2002) of the Food and Nutrition Board of the National Academies of Sciences, Engineering, and Medicine. She received the Fomon Nutrition Award from the American Academy of Pediatrics and is a fellow of the American Society of Nutrition.

Mary Story, Ph.D., R.D., is a professor in Community and Family Medicine and Global Health and also serves as the associate director for academic programs in the Duke Global Institute. She brings to this position 13 years serving in leadership positions at the University of Minnesota School of Public Health, including as senior associate dean for academic and student affairs at the school from 2011 to 2013. Dr. Story is a leading scholar in the field of child and adolescent nutrition and child obesity prevention and has published more than 400 scientific articles. Dr. Story has devoted her research career to the study of child and adolescent nutrition and childhood obesity. Her research has focused primarily on nutrition and diet-related issues of low-income and minority youth and their families, and environmental and behavioral community-based obesity prevention interventions for youth. Dr. Story has conducted several National Institutes of Health–funded school and community-based obesity prevention trials. Since 2005, Dr. Story has directed the Healthy Eating Research program, a national program of the Robert Wood Johnson Foundation that supports research on environmental and policy strategies to promote healthy eating among children to prevent childhood obesity. She was elected to the National Academy of Medicine in 2010.

Margo Wootan, D.Sc., is the director of nutrition policy at the Center for Science in the Public Interest (CSPI), one of the country's leading health advocacy organizations that specializes in food, nutrition, and obesity prevention. Dr. Wootan received her B.S. degree in nutrition from Cornell University and her D.Sc. in nutrition from Harvard University's School of Public Health. She co-founded and coordinates the activities of the National Alliance for Nutrition and Activity (NANA) and the Food Marketing Workgroup. She has coordinated and led efforts to require calorie labeling at fast-food and other chain restaurants, require trans fat labeling on packaged foods, improve school foods, reduce junk-food marketing aimed at children, and expand nutrition and physical activity programs at the Centers for Disease Control and Prevention. Dr. Wootan has received numerous awards and is quoted regularly in the nation's major media.

Appendix C

Bibliography of References Used to Inform Workshop Planning[1]

DIETARY INTAKE, FEEDING PRACTICES, AND TASTE PREFERENCES OF YOUNG CHILDREN

Birch, L. L., and A. E. Doub. 2014. Learning to eat: Birth to age 2 y. *American Journal of Clinical Nutrition* 99(3):723S–728S.

Deming, D. M., R. R. Briefel, and K. C. Reidy. 2014. Infant feeding practices and food consumption patterns of children participating in WIC. *Journal of Nutrition Education and Behavior* 46(3 Suppl):S29–S37.

Ford, C. N., S. W. Ng, and B. M. Popkin. 2016. Ten-year beverage intake trends among U.S. preschool children: Rapid declines between 2003 and 2010 but stagnancy in recent years. *Pediatric Obesity* 11(1):47–53.

Gandarvaka, M., and A. M. Siega-Riz. 2017. Trends in food and beverage consumption among infants and toddlers: 2005–2012. *Pediatrics* 139(6):e20163290.

Grimes, C. A., E. A. Szymlek-Gay, and T. A. Nicklas. 2017. Beverage consumption among U.S. children ages 0-24 months: National Health and Nutrition Examination Survey (NHANES). *Nutrients* 9(3):e264.

Mennella, J. A. 2014. Ontogeny of taste preferences: Basic biology and implications for health. *American Journal of Clinical Nutrition* 99(3):704S–711S.

Park, S., L. Pan, B. Sherry, and R. Li. 2014. The association of sugar-sweetened beverage intake during infancy with sugar-sweetened beverage intake at 6 years of age. *Pediatrics* 134(Suppl 1):S56–S62.

Park, S., R. Li, and L. Birch. 2015. Mothers' child-feeding practices are associated with children's sugar-sweetened beverage intake. *Journal of Nutrition* 145(4):806–812.

Rosinger, A., K. Herrick, J. Gahche, and S. Park. 2017. Sugar-sweetened beverage consumption among U.S. youth, 2011–2014. *NCHS Data Brief* (271):1–8.

[1] This list was provided as a handout at the workshop.

GUIDELINES, ADVISORY REPORTS, AND SCIENTIFIC STATEMENTS

Abrams, S. A., and S. R. Daniels. 2017. Fruit juice and child health. *Pediatrics* 139(4):e20170041.

Council on School Health, Committee on Nutrition. 2015. Snacks, sweetened beverages, added sugars, and schools. *Pediatrics* 135(3):575–583.

Heyman, M. B., S. A. Abrams, and the American Academy of Pediatrics Section on Gastroenterology, Hepatology, and Nutrition, Committee on Nutrition. 2017. Fruit juice in infants, children, and adolescents: Current recommendations. *Pediatrics* e20170967.

HHS/USDA (U.S. Department of Health and Human Services/U.S. Department of Agriculture). 2015. *Dietary Guidelines for Americans 2015–2020: Eighth edition*. https://health.gov/dietaryguidelines/2015/guidelines (accessed June 20, 2017).

HHS/USDA. 2015. *Scientific report of the 2015 Dietary Guidelines Advisory Committee*. Washington, DC: Agricultural Research Service, U.S. Department of Agriculture.

Pérez-Escamilla, R., S. Segura-Pérez, M. Lott, on behalf of the Robert Wood Johnson Foundation Healthy Eating Research Expert Panel on Best Practices for Promoting Healthy Nutrition, Feeding Patterns, and Weight Status for Infants and Toddlers from Birth to 24 Months. 2017. *Feeding guidelines for infants and young toddlers: A responsive parenting approach*. Durham, NC: Healthy Eating Research.

Vos, M. B., J. L. Kaar, J. A. Welsh, L. V. Van Horn, D. I. Feig, C. A. M. Anderson, M. J. Patel, J. Cruz Munos, N. F. Krebs, S. A. Xanthakos, R. K. Johnson, American Heart Association Nutrition Committee of the Council on Lifestyle and Cardiometabolic Health, Council on Clinical Cardiology, Council on Cardiovascular Disease in the Young, Council on Cardiovascular and Stroke Nursing, Council on Epidemiology and Prevention, Council on Functional Genomics and Translational Biology, and Council on Hypertension. 2017. Added sugars and cardiovascular disease risk in children: A scientific statement from the American Heart Association. *Circulation* 135(19):e1017–e1034.

SELECT APPROACHES, INTERVENTIONS, AND TOOLKITS

Boles, M., A. Adams, A. Gredler, and S. Manhas. 2014. Ability of a mass media campaign to influence knowledge, attitudes, and behaviors about sugary drinks and obesity. *Preventive Medicine* 67(Suppl 1):S40–S45.

CDC (Centers for Disease Control and Prevention). 2015. *Food service guidelines: Case studies states and communities*. Atlanta, GA: U.S. Department of Health and Human Services.

CDC. 2017. Nutrition: Strategies and resources. https://www.cdc.gov/nccdphp/dnpao/state-local-programs/nutrition.html (accessed June 20, 2017).

Center for Science in the Public Interest. 2017. *The national movement to improve restaurant children's meals*. http://www.foodmarketing.org/wp-content/uploads/2017/04/NationalMovement.pdf (accessed June 20, 2017).

ChangeLab Solutions. 2013. *Sugar-sweetened beverages playbook: 10 strategies to reduce SSB consumption*. http://www.changelabsolutions.org/publications/SSB-playbook (accessed June 20, 2017).

Cradock, A. L., J. L. Barrett, E. L. Kenney, C. M. Giles, Z. J. Ward, M. W. Long, S. C. Resch, A. A. Pipito, E. R. Wei, and S. L. Gortmaker. 2017. Using cost-effectiveness analysis to prioritize policy and programmatic approaches to physical activity promotion and obesity prevention in childhood. *Preventive Medicine* 95(Suppl):S17–S27.

de Ruyter, J. C., M. R. Olthof, J. C. Seidell, and M. B. Katan. 2012. A trial of sugar-free or sugar-sweetened beverages and body weight in children. *New England Journal of Medicine* 367(15):1397–1406.

Gortmaker, S. L., Y. C. Wang, M. W. Long, C. M. Giles, Z. J. Ward, J. L. Barrett, E. L. Kenney, K. R. Sonneville, A. S. Afzal, S. C. Resch, and A. L. Cradock. 2015. Three interventions that reduce childhood obesity are projected to save more than they cost to implement. *Health Affairs (Millwood)* 34(11):1932–1939.

Horizon Foundation. 2017. *Howard County Unsweetened.* http://www.hocounsweetened.org (accessed June 20, 2017).

Indian Health Services. 2013. *Healthy beverages community action guide.* https://www.ihs.gov/nutrition/includes/themes/newihstheme/display_objects/documents/HealthyBeverages508.pdf (accessed June 20, 2017).

Kansagra, S. M., M. O. Kennelly, C. A. Nonas, C. J. Curtis, G. Van Wye, A. Goodman, and T. A. Farley. Reducing sugary drink consumption: New York City's approach. *American Journal of Public Health* 105(4):e61–e64.

Lederer, A., C. J. Curtis, L. D. Silver, and S. Y. Angell. 2014. Toward a healthier city: Nutrition standards for New York City government. *American Journal of Preventive Medicine* 46(4):423–428.

Roberto, C. A., D. Wong, A. Musicus, and D. Hammond. 2016. The influence of sugar-sweetened beverage health warning labels on parents' choices. *Pediatrics* 137(2):e20153185.

Schwartz, A. E., M. Leardo, S. Aneja, and B. Elbel. 2016. Effect of a school-based water intervention on child body mass index and obesity. *JAMA Pediatrics* 170(3):220–226.

Schwartz, M. B., G. E. Schneider, Y. Y. Choi, X. Li, J. Harris, T. Andreyeva, M. Hyary, N. Highsmith Vernick, and L. J. Appel. 2017. Association of a community campaign for better beverage choices with beverage purchases from supermarkets. *JAMA Internal Medicine* 177(5):666–674.

VanEpps, E. M., and C. A. Roberto. 2016. The influence of sugar-sweetened beverage warnings: A randomized trial of adolescents' choices and beliefs. *American Journal of Preventive Medicine* 51(5):664–672.

Voices for Healthy Kids. 2017. *Fact sheet—Healthy restaurant children's meals improve diets and health.* http://kidsmeals.voicesforhealthykids.org/resources/fact-sheet-healthy-restaurant-childrens-meals-improve-diets-and-health (accessed June 20, 2017).

EARLY CHILD CARE AND EDUCATION SETTINGS

Breck, A., K. Goodman, L. Dunn, R. L. Stephens, N. Dawkins, B. Dixon, J. Jernigan, J. Kakietek, C. Lesesne, L. Lessard, C. Nonas, S. A. O'Dell, T. A. Osuji, B. Bronson, Y. Xu, and L. Kettel Khan. 2014. Evaluation design of New York City's regulations on nutrition, physical activity, and screen time in early child care centers. *Preventing Chronic Disease* 11:E184.

CDC (Centers for Disease Control and Prevention). 2014. *Increasing access to drinking water and other healthier beverages in early care and education settings.* Atlanta, GA: U.S. Department of Health and Human Services.

CDC. 2016. *Early care and education state indicator report.* Atlanta, GA: U.S. Department of Health and Human Services.

Kakietek, J., T. A. Osuji, S. A. O'Dell, A. Breck, and L. Kettel Khan. 2014. Compliance with New York City's beverage regulations and beverage consumption among children in early child care centers. *Preventing Chronic Disease* 16(11):E180.

Lessard, L., C. Lesesne, J. Kakietek, A. Breck, J. Jernigan, L. Dunn, C. Nonas, S. A. O'Dell, R. L. Stephens, Y. Xu, and L. Kettel Khan. 2014. Measurement of compliance with New York City's regulations on beverages, physical activity, and screen time in early child care centers. *Preventing Chronic Disease* 11:E183.

Nanney, M. S., T. L. LaRowe, C. Davey, N. Frost, C. Arcan, and J. O'Meara. 2017. Obesity prevention in early child care settings. *Health Education and Behavior* 44(1):23–31.

Sekhobo, J. P., L. S. Edmunds, K. Dalenius, J. Jernigan, C. F. Davis, M. Giddings, C. Lesesne, and L. Kettel Khan. Neighborhood disparities in prevalence of childhood obesity among low-income children before and after implementation of New York City child care regulations. *Preventing Chronic Disease* 11:E181.

Ward, D. S., S. E. Benjamin, A. S. Ammerman, S. C. Ball, B. H. Neelon, and S. I. Bangdiwala. 2008. Nutrition and physical activity in child care: Results from an environmental intervention. *American Journal of Preventive Medicine* 35(4):352–356.

NUTRITION ASSISTANCE PROGRAMS

Andreyeva, T., J. Luedicke, A. S. Tripp, and K. E. Henderson. 2013. Effects of reduced juice allowances in food packages for the Women, Infants, and Children program. *Pediatrics* 131(5):919–927.

Andreyeva, T., A. S. Tripp, and M. B. Schwartz. 2015. Dietary quality of Americans by Supplemental Nutrition Assistance Program participation status: A systematic review. *American Journal of Preventive Medicine* 49(4):594–604.

Barnhill, A. 2011. Impact and ethics of excluding sweetened beverages from the SNAP program. *American Journal of Public Health* 101(11):2037–2043.

Chrisinger, B. W. 2017. Ethical imperatives against item restriction in the Supplemental Nutrition Assistance Program. *Preventive Medicine* 100:56–60.

Grummon, A. H., and L. S. Taillie. 2017. Nutritional profile of Supplemental Nutrition Assistance Program household food and beverage purchases. *American Journal of Clinical Nutrition* 105(6):1433–1442.

Harnack, L., J. M. Oakes, B. Elbel, T. Beatty, S. Rydell, and S. French. 2016. Effects of subsidies and prohibitions on nutrition in a food benefit program: A randomized clinical trial. *JAMA Internal Medicine* 176(11):1610–1618.

Kennedy, E., and J. F. Guthrie. 2016. Nutrition assistance programs: Cause or solution to obesity. *Current Obesity Reports* 5(2):176–183.

Liu, J., T. Kuo, L. Jiang, B. Robles, and S. E. Whaley. 2016. Food and drink consumption among 1–5-year-old Los Angeles County children from households receiving dual SNAP and WIC v. only WIC benefits. *Public Health Nutrition* 1–8.

Nguyen, B. T., and L. M. Powell. 2015. Supplemental Nutrition Assistance Program participation and sugar-sweetened beverage consumption, overall and by source. *Preventive Medicine* 81:82–86.

Pomeranz, J. L., and J. F. Chriqui. 2015. The Supplemental Nutrition Assistance Program: Analysis of program administration and food law definitions. *American Journal of Preventive Medicine* 49(3):428–436.

Schwartz, M. B. 2017. Moving beyond the debate over restricting sugary drinks in the Supplemental Nutrition Assistance Program. *American Journal of Preventive Medicine* 52(2S2):S199–S205.

Watowicz, R. P., and C. A. Taylor. 2014. A comparison of beverage intakes in U.S. children based on WIC participation and eligibility. *Journal of Nutrition Education and Behavior* 46(3 Suppl):S59–S64.

LOCAL ORDINANCES AND LEGAL CONSIDERATIONS

City of Perris, California. 2017. *Council approves healthy drink ordinance.* http://www.cityofperris.org/news/2017/stories/03-21-17_healthy-drink.html (accessed June 20, 2017).

Davis, California, Municipal Code § 17.02.

Gostin, L. O., B. H. Reeve, and M. Ashe. 2014. The historic role of boards of health in local innovation: New York City's soda portion case. *JAMA* 312(15):1511–1512.

Pomeranz, J. L., and M. Pertschuk. 2017. State preemption: A significant and quiet threat to public health in the United States. *American Journal of Public Health* 107(6):900–902.

Roberto, C. A., and J. L. Pomeranz. 2015. Public health and legal arguments in favor of a policy to cap the portion sizes of sugar-sweetened beverages. *American Journal of Public Health* 105(11):2183–2190.

Stockton, California, Municipal Code § 5.70.

Studdert, D. M., J. Flanders, and M. M. Mello. 2015. Searching for public health law's sweet spot: The regulation of sugar-sweetened beverages. *PLoS Medicine* 12(7):e1001848.

TAXATION

Barrientos-Gutierrez. T., R. Zepeda-Tello, E. R. Rodrigues, A. Colchero-Aragonés, R. Rojas-Martínez, E. Lazcano-Ponce, M. Hernández-Ávila, J. Rivera-Dommarco, and R. Meza. 2017. Expected population weight and diabetes impact of the 1-peso-per-litre tax to sugar sweetened beverages in Mexico. *PLoS ONE* 12(5):e0176336.

Colchero, M. A., B. M. Popkin, J. A. Rivera, and S. W. Ng. 2016. Beverage purchases from stores in Mexico under the excise tax on sugar sweetened beverages: Observational study. *BMJ* 352:h6704.

Falbe, J., N. Rojas, A. H. Grummon, and K. A. Madsen. 2015. Higher retail prices of sugar-sweetened beverages 3 months after implementation of an excise tax in Berkeley, California. *American Journal of Public Health* 105(11):2194–2201.

Falbe, J., H. R. Thompson, C. M. Becker, N. Rojas, C. E. McCulloch, and K. A. Madsen. 2016. Impact of the Berkeley excise tax on sugar-sweetened beverage consumption. *American Journal of Public Health* 106(10):1865–1871.

Public Health Institute. 2017. Berkeley's sugar sweetened beverage tax: What happened to jobs and business revenue? http://www.phi.org/uploads/application/files/zq8houfhy138b4rggefjpaj7t2s7k2hpjfpjofgin6pw2tp77h.pdf (accessed June 20, 2017).

Silver, L. D., S. W. Ng, S. Ryan-Ibarra, L. S. Taillie, M. Induni, D. R. Miles, J. M. Poti, and B. M. Popkin. 2017. Changes in prices, sales, consumer spending, and beverage consumption one year after a tax on sugar-sweetened beverages in Berkeley, California, U.S.: A before-and-after study. *PLoS Medicine* 14(4):e1002283.

THE ROLE OF INDUSTRY

Better Business Bureau. 2017. *Children's food & beverage advertising initiatives.* http://www.bbb.org/council/the-national-partner-program/national-advertising-review-services/childrens-food-and-beverage-advertising-initiative (accessed June 20, 2017).

Emond, J. A., M. E. Smith, S. J. Mathur, J. D. Sargent, and D. Gilbert-Diamond. 2015. Children's food and beverage promotion on television to parents. *Pediatrics* 136(6):1095–1102.

Harris, J. L., M. B. Schwartz, M. LoDolce, C. Munsell, F. Fleming-Milici, J. Elsey, S. Liu, M. Hyary, R. Gross, C. Hazen, and C. Dembek. 2014. Sugary drink FACTS 2014: Some progress but much room for improvement in marking to youth. Hartford, CT: Rudd Center for Food Policy and Obesity.

Harris, J. L., F. Fleming-Milici, W. Frazier, H. Haraghey, S. Kalnova, M. Romo-Palafox, N. Seymour, G. Rodriguez-Arauz, and M. B. Schwartz. 2017. Baby food FACTS: Nutrition and marking of baby and toddler food and drink. Hartford, CT: Rudd Center for Food Policy and Obesity.

Keybridge. 2016a. *2025 Beverage Calories Initiative: 2015 Progress on the national initiative.* http://keybridgedc.com/wp-content/uploads/2017/05/2025-Beverage-Calories-Initiative_National-Initiative_2015-Progress.pdf (accessed June 20, 2017).

Keybridge. 2016b. *2025 Beverage Calories Initiative: Baseline report for the national initiative.* http://keybridgedc.com/wp-content/uploads/2016/04/2025-Beverage-Calories-Initiative_National-Initiative_Baseline-Report.pdf (accessed June 20, 2017).

Kraak, V. I., and M. Story. 2015. Guiding principles and a decision-making framework for stakeholders pursuing healthy food environments. *Health Affairs* 34(11):1972–1978.

Munsell, C. R., J. L. Harris, V. Sarda, and M. B. Schwartz. 2016. Parents' beliefs about the healthfulness of sugary drink options: Opportunities to address misperceptions. *Public Health Nutrition* 19(1):46–54.

Nixon, L., P. Mejia, A. Cheyne, C. Wilking, L. Dorfman, and R. Daynard. 2015. "We're part of the solution": Evolution of the food and beverage industry's framing of obesity concerns between 2000 and 2012. *American Journal of Public Health* 105(11):2228–2236.

Powell, L. M., R. M. Schermbeck, and F. J. Chaloupka. 2013. Nutritional content of food and beverage products in television advertisements seen on children's programming. *Childhood Obesity* 9(6):524–531.

Scott, C., B. Hawkins, and C. Knai. 2017. Food and beverage product reformulation as a corporate political strategy. *Social Science and Medicine* 172:37–45.

Wescott, R. F., B. M. Fitzpatrick, and E. Phillips. 2012. Industry self-regulation to improve student health: Quantifying changes in beverage shipments to schools. *American Journal of Public Health* 102(10):1928–1935.

Wescott, R. F., B. Fitzpatrick, and E. Phillips. 2015. *2014 Progress report, McDonald's-Alliance for a Healthier Generation partnership: Clinton Global Initiative commitment to action.* http://keybridgedc.com/wp-content/uploads/2015/06/2014-Progress-Report_McDonalds-Alliance-Partnership-on-CGI-Commitment-to-Action-06-25-15.pdf (accessed June 20, 2017).